Student Laboratory Manual for

Physical Examination and Health Assessment

Second Edition

CAROLYN JARVIS, RN, C, MSN, FNP

Adjunct Assistant Professor
School of Nursing
Illinois Wesleyan University
Bloomington, Illinois
and
Family Nurse Practitioner
Chestnut Health Systems
Bloomington, Illinois

W.B. SAUNDERS COMPANY
A Division of Harcourt Brace & Company
Philadelphia London Toronto Montreal Sydney Tokyo

W. B. Saunders Company
A Division of Harcourt Brace & Company
The Curtis Center
Independence Square West
Philadelphia, PA 19106-3399

Student Laboratory Manual for
PHYSICAL EXAMINATION AND HEALTH ASSESSMENT
Second Edition

ISBN 0-7216-5986-1

Printed in the United States of America

Last digit is the print number: 9   8   7   6   5

Preface

This Lab Manual is intended as a study guide and laboratory manual to accompany the textbook *Physical Examination and Health Assessment*, 2nd edition. You will use it in two places: in your own study area, and in the skills laboratory.

As a study guide, this workbook highlights and reinforces the content from the text. Each chapter corresponds to a chapter in the textbook and contains workbook exercises and questions in varying formats that provide the repetition needed to synthesize and master content from the text. Fill out the lab manual chapter and answer the questions before coming to the skills laboratory. This will reinforce your lectures, expose any areas needing questioning for your clinical instructor, and prime you for the skills laboratory/clinical experience.

Once in the skills laboratory, use the Lab Manual as a direct clinical tool. Each chapter contains assessment forms on perforated tear-out pages. Usually you will work in pairs and perform the regional physical examinations on each other under the tutelage of your instructor. As you perform the examination on your peer, you can fill out the write-up sheet and assessment form to be handed in and checked by the instructor.

FEATURES

Each chapter is divided into two parts, cognitive and clinical, and contains:

- Purpose—a brief summary of the material you are learning in this chapter
- Reading Assignment—the corresponding chapter and page numbers from the textbook, and space for your instructor to assign journal articles
- Audio-Visual Assignment—space for your instructor to assign relevant videos, audio tapes, or computer-assisted learning modules
- Glossary—important and specialized terms from the textbook chapter with accompanying definitions
- Study Guide—specific short answer and fill in questions to help you highlight and learn content from the chapter. Important art figures of human anatomy have been reproduced from the textbook with the labels deleted so that you can identify and fill in the names of the structures yourself.
- Review Questions—multiple choice, matching, and short answer questions in a format similar to usual college classroom exams, so that you can monitor your own mastery of the material. Take the self-exam when you are ready and then check your answers with the correct answers given in Appendix A.
- Clinical Objectives—behavioral objectives that you should achieve during your peer practice in the regional examinations
- Regional write-up sheets—complete yet succinct physical examination forms that you can use in the skills lab or in the clinical setting. These serve as a memory prompt, listing key history questions and physical exam steps, and they serve as a means of recording data during the client encounter.
- Narrative summary forms— S O A P format, so that you can learn to chart narrative accounts of the history and physical exam findings. These forms have accompanying sketches of regional anatomy, and are an especially useful exercise for those studying for advanced practice roles.

Learning the skills of history taking and physical examination requires two kinds of practice, cognitive and clinical. It is my hope that this Student Laboratory Manual will help you achieve both of these learning and practice modalities.

Carolyn Jarvis

Acknowledgment

I am grateful to many people who helped make this Laboratory Manual a reality. I am grateful to Helen Noyes Downey who contributed the well composed and challenging review questions for each chapter and to Joyce Keithley who submitted the glossary for the nutrition chapter. At W. B. Saunders Company, my thanks extend to: Barbara Nelson Cullen, Senior Acquisitions Editor, for her unflagging support and decisive leadership on this project; Alison Zaintz, The Production House, Inc., for her professional shaping of typed manuscript into camera ready copy, and, finally, to Francine Rosenthal, Assistant Developmental Editor, for her skillful and cheerful guidance in shepherding the manual from start to finish. Back at the home office, I am grateful to Marcie Tempel for her help in library sleuthing, to Julia Jarvis for office assistance, and to Sarah Jarvis for her help in typing many of the early chapters.

Contents

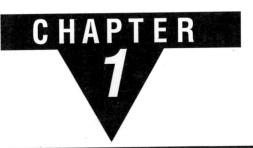

Assessment for Health and Illness

Purpose: This chapter introduces the concept of health including the evolving definition of health through the twentieth century; helps you to understand that it is the definition of health that determines the kinds of factors that are assessed; and shows you that the amount of data gathered during assessment varies with the person's age, developmental state, physical condition, risk factors, and culture.

Reading Assignment: Jarvis, *Physical Examination and Health Assessment*, 2nd ed., Chapter 1, pp. 4-10

Glossary: Study the following terms after reading the corresponding chapter in the text. You should be able to cover the definition on the right and define the term out loud.

Assessment .... the collection of data about an individual's health state

Biomedical model.................... the Western European/North American tradition that views health as the absence of disease

Complete data base.................. a complete health history and full physical examination

Emergency data base .... rapid collection of the data base, often compiled concurrently with lifesaving measures

Environment .... the total of all the conditions and elements that make up the surroundings and influence the development of a person

Episodic data base .... one used for a limited or short-term problem; concerns mainly one problem, one cue complex, or one body system

Follow-up data base .... used in all settings to monitor progress on short-term or chronic health problems

Holistic health.......................... the view that the mind, body, and spirit are interdependent and function as a whole within the environment

Medical diagnosis.................... used to evaluate the cause and etiology of disease; focus is on the function or malfunction of a specific organ system

Nursing diagnosis .... used to evaluate the response of the whole person to actual or potential health problems

Objective data .... what the health professional observes by inspecting, palpating, percussing, and auscultating during the physical examination

Prevention .... any action directed toward promoting health and preventing the occurrence of disease

Subjective data .... what the person says about himself or herself during history taking

Wellness .... a dynamic process and view of health; a move toward optimal functioning

STUDY GUIDE

After completing the reading assignment you should be able to answer the following questions in the spaces provided.

1. Relate each of the following concepts of health to the process of data collection:

    biomedical model

    wellness

    holistic health

    prevention.

2. Differentiate *subjective* data from *objective* data by placing an S or O after each of the following: complaint of sore shoulder _S_ ; unconscious _O_ ; blood in the urine _O_ ; family has just moved to a new area _S_ ; dizziness _O_ ; sore throat _O_ ; earache _O_ ; weight gain _O_ .

3. How are medical diagnosis and nursing diagnosis similar?

    How are they different?

4. For the following situations, state the type of data collection you would perform (i.e., *complete* data base, *episodic* or problem centered data base, *follow up* data base, *emergency* data base). Barbiturate overdose ___EMERGENCY___; ambulatory, apparently well individual who presents at outpatient clinic with a rash___EPISODIC___; first visit to a health care provider for a "checkup"___COMPLETE___; recently placed on antihypertensive medication ___FOLLOWUP___.

5. Discuss the term *minority* as it applies to culturally diverse individuals.

6. List 3 health care interactions you have experienced yourself with another person from a culture or ethnicity different from your own. You may have been the patient or the provider—it makes no difference.

7. Using one sentence or group of phrases, how would you describe your own health state to someone you are meeting for the first time?

   I FEEL GOOD.
   I AM PHYSICALLY AND MENTALLY OF GOOD HEALTH.

8. Considering your own health state, how would you describe yourself (brief phrase or phrases) in each of the following assessment factors:

   Growth and development _____

   Biophysical status _____

   Emotional status _____

   Cultural, religious, socioeconomic background _____

   _____

   Performance of activities of daily living _____

   _____

Patterns of coping _____

Interaction patterns _____

Satisfaction with your health state _____

Your health goals _____

Environment (physical, social, emotional, ecological) _____

_____

_____

Accessible human and material resources _____

_____

REVIEW QUESTIONS

This test is for you and is intended to check your own mastery of the content. Answers are provided in Appendix A.

1. The concept of health has expanded in the past 40 years. Select the term that reflects the most narrow description of health.

   a) the absence of disease
   b) a dynamic process toward optimal functioning
   c) depends on an interaction of mind, body, and spirit within the environment
   d) prevention of disease

2. Select the most complete description of a data base.

   a) subjective and objective data gathered by a health practitioner from a client
   b) objective data obtained from a client through inspection, percussion, palpation, and auscultation
   c) a summary of a client's record including laboratory studies
   d) subjective and objective data gathered from a client plus the results of any diagnostic studies completed

3. Nursing diagnoses, based on assessment of a number of factors, give nurses a common language with which to communicate nursing findings. The best description of a nursing diagnosis is:

   a) used to evaluate the etiology of a disease
   b) a judgment about the health status of an individual
   c) a concise, problem-centered description of actual or potential health problems that alter one's life processes
   d) an efficient basis for communicating client data among nurses both intra and inter agency

4. Depending on the clinical situation, the nurse may establish one of four kinds of data base. An episodic data base is described as:

   a) including a complete health history and full physical examination.
   b) concerning mainly one problem.
   c) evaluation of a previously identified problem.
   d) rapid collection of data in conjunction with lifesaving measures.

5. Individuals should be seen at regular intervals for health care. The frequency of these visits:

   a) is most efficient if performed on an annual basis.
   b) is not important. There is no recommendation for the frequency of health care.
   c) varies, depending upon the age of the client.
   d) is based on the practitioner's clinical experience.

6. Cultural diversity is currently considered when discussing health assessment and care. From a nursing perspective, the most accurate description of this phenomenon is:

   a) nursing is inherently a transcultural phenomenon. The process of helping people involves at least two people having different cultural orientations.
   b) a consideration when the nurse is caring for someone identified as a minority among the local population.
   c) the consideration of the needs of 51.1 percent of the population of the United States that do not have European ancestry.
   d) an area that has always been of consideration to nursing and is included in most nursing curricula.

7. Briefly summarize the concepts discussed in the chapter titled *Assessment of the Whole Person.*

CHAPTER 2

Developmental Tasks and Health Promotion Across the Life Cycle

Purpose: This chapter gives a general portrayal of the individual in each stage of the life cycle considering the physical, psychosocial, cognitive, and behavioral development of the person; presents age specific charts for periodic health examination that detail the screening examination measures, counseling for health promotion, and risk factors for each age group; and presents a few developmental screening tests used in clinical practice.

Reading Assignment: Jarvis, *Physical Examination and Health Assessment*, 2nd ed., Chapter 2, pp. 11-46

Glossary: Study the following terms after reading the corresponding chapter in the text. You should be able to cover the definition on the right and define the term out loud.

Centration	the characteristic of focusing on only one aspect of a situation at a time and ignoring other characteristics
Cooperative play	children playing the same game and interacting while doing it
Delayed imitation	a child can witness an event, form a mental representation of it, and imitate it later in the absence of the model
Egocentric	the characteristic of focusing on one's own interests, needs, and point of view and lacking concern for others
Latency	Freud's term for the relative sexual quiet of the time of middle childhood
Mental representation	Piaget's term for the concept acquired by age 2 that an infant can think of an external event without actually experiencing it
Object permanence	Piaget's term for the concept acquired during infancy that objects and people continue to exist even when they are no longer in sight
Prehension	using the hand and fingers for the act of grasping
Stress	the total of the biologic reactions to an adverse stimulus—whether it be physical, mental, or emotional, internal or external—that tends to disturb the homeostasis of the body
Symbolic function	Piaget's term for the concept acquired during childhood in which the child uses symbols to represent people, objects, and events

Telegraphic speech .... speech used by age 3 or 4 in which three- or four-word sentences contain only the essential words

Transductive reasoning .... the young child's thinking that when two events occur simultaneously, that one caused the other, even though they are unrelated

STUDY GUIDE

After completing the reading assignment, you should be able to answer the following questions in the spaces provided.

1. List 9 developmental stages, from infancy through late adulthood, and give the general age ranges for each stage.

2. List Erikson's 8 stages of ego development that encompass the life span, and state the distinct conflict, or *crisis*, that characterizes each stage.

3. List Piaget's stages of cognitive development in the growing child and state the way of thinking that characterizes each stage.

4. List at least 4 points of parent counseling that you should include on a periodic health examination for an infant, age birth to 18 months (see Table 2 - 1, p. 15 in Jarvis, *Physical Examination and Health Assessment, 2nd ed.*).

5. Define toddler lordosis.

6. State 4 points of physical examination screening you should perform during a young child's periodic health examination, ages 2 - 6.

7. The preadolescent growth spurt occurs at about age _____ in girls and about age _____ in boys.

8. State at least 6 points of patient and parent counseling you should include during the periodic health examination for the middle childhood years, ages 7–12.

9. List at least 4 developmental tasks that characterize the stage of adolescence.

10. List the points of counseling for substance use, sexual practices, and injury prevention that you would include during patient teaching in the periodic health examination of an adolescent, ages 13–18.

11. State the 5 leading causes of death for adult years, ages 19–39.

12. List 5 items of physical examination aimed at screening certain high risk groups during a periodic health examination on a younger adult, ages 19 - 39.

13. State the frequency with which the following tests of physical examination should be performed on a middle aged adult, ages 40 - 64.

    Clinical breast examination for women _____

    Papanicolaou smear for women _____

    Auscultation for carotid bruits _____

    Influenza vaccine for those at risk _____

14. State the 6 leading causes of death for older adults, ages 65 and over.

15. List the screening laboratory/diagnostic procedures that should be performed yearly on older adults ages 65 and over.

16. Discuss the implications of conducting a life review, which is one of the developmental tasks confronting older adults.

Note that 6 tables summarizing growth and development milestones for infancy through adolescence can be found in the appendices of this Laboratory Manual, for your reference.

REVIEW QUESTIONS

This test is for you and is intended to check your own mastery of the content. Answers are provided in Appendix A.

1. Select the best description of the physical growth of an average term infant during the first year of life.

   a) between 5 and 7 pounds at birth. Weight and height double by 1 year.

   b) between 5 1/2 and 10 pounds at birth. Weight and height triple by 1 year

   c) between 5 1/2 and 10 pounds at birth. Weight triples and height doubles by 1 year.

   d) 7 1/2 pounds at birth. Weight and height double by 1 year.

2. Human development has been studied by a number of theorists. The best description of Erik Erikson's theory is that it is:

   a) concerned with biologic determinants of behavior.

   b) concerned with the growth of the ego.

   c) concerned with cognitive development in the growing child

   d) concerned with physiologic development from infancy to 1 year.

3. A game of hide and seek is an example of:

   a) Piaget's object permanence.

   b) Levinson's settling down.

   c) Freud's biologic determinant of behavior.

   d) Erikson's theory of trust versus mistrust.

4. B. D., age 15 months, has come to the clinic for a well baby visit. This is the first visit for this child since the family recently relocated. When a developmental history is taken from the mother she states "Beth just started to pull herself up to a standing position." The best action on the part of the practitioner is to:

   a) proceed with the exam. The child is progressing at the expected rate.

   b) proceed with the exam. Although the child is behind the anticipated developmental stage, the child is clearly progressing in a cephalocaudal direction.

   c) perform a complete examination, focusing on the musculoskeletal system. Then discuss the findings with the mother.

   d) obtain a more detailed physical development history, then perform the examination. This represents a developmental delay for this child.

5. The use of two-word phrases by a 2-year-old is an example of:

   a) biphrase.
   b) holophrase.
   c) telegraphic speech.
   d) ritualism.

6. Screening for amblyopia and strabismus should be part of the periodic health examination for a child:

   a) birth to 18 months
   b) 2–6 years of age.
   c) 7–12 years of age.
   d) 13–18 years of age.

7. A group of children are observed playing a game. The observer would recognize this as:

   a) parallel play.
   b) language development.
   c) decentration.
   d) cooperative play.

8. During a periodic health visit, the practitioner discusses the use of bicycle safety helmets. This would be most appropriate for children:

   a) birth to 18 months
   b) 2 - 6 years of age.
   c) 7 - 12 years of age.
   d) 13 - 18 years of age.

9. As with other age groups, the periodic health examination for children ages 13 to 18 includes screening for for various risks. A complete skin assessment for this group would:

   a) be part of the scheduled screening.
   b) be completed only for high risk groups.
   c) not usually be included with this age group. Should be included for 7–12 year olds.
   d) be completed to provide early intervention for acne.

10. The description of alternative periods of structure building and transition in an adult's life are the results of the work of:

   a) Erik Erikson
   b) Sigmund Freud
   c) Gail Sheehy
   d) Daniel Levinson

11. A life review or taking stock is usually associated with the developmental period of

   a) early adulthood.
   b) middle adulthood.
   c) late adulthood.
   d) late, late adulthood.

SKILLS LABORATORY/ CLINICAL SETTING

   You are now ready for the clinical component of mastering the content in this chapter. The purpose of the clinical component is to practice administering the developmental screening tests on a volunteer or a peer and gain some comfort with the tool before administering it on clients of your own.

   The Denver II is a screening instrument designed to detect developmental delays in infants and preschoolers, and is described in more detail in Jarvis, *Physical Examination and Health Assessment, 2nd ed.*, pp. 37–40. Study the text and make certain you are familiar with the tool. The Denver II was carefully standardized with very specific instructions for the administration and interpretation of each item. These are contained in the Denver II Training Manual.In addition to the instrument, you will need a kit of items (yarn, cube, doll, etc.) that are used during the test. Also, you will need a healthy young child on whom to practice. Perhaps a classmate or a faculty member can volunteer his or her young child for one administration of the test.

   The Recent Life Changes Questionnarie is a tool that attempts to quantify the impact of life change and life stress on an adult's health. You should take this questionnaire yourself. Be aware that some of the questions are sensitive and considered personal by many people. You should be aware of this when considering whether or not to discuss your own questionnaire with your classmate or faculty member. You will gain considerable insight in taking the test, both on the impact of life change on adults, and on the amount of life change occuring in your own life.

NOTES

RECENT LIFE CHANGES QUESTIONNAIRE

I. INSTRUCTIONS FOR MARKING YOUR RECENT CHANGES

To answer the questions below, mark an "X" in one or more of the columns to the right of each question. If the event in question has occurred to you within the past two years, indicate when it occurred by marking the appropriate column: 0–6 months ago, 7–12 months ago, etc. It may be the case with some of the events below that you experienced them over more than one of the time periods listed for the past two years. If so, mark all of the appropriate columns. If the event has not occurred to you during the last two years (or has never occurred to you) leave all the columns empty.

Now go through the questionnaire and mark your recent life changes. The column marked "Your Adjustment Score" will be explained at the end of the questionnaire.

A. HEALTH

Within the time periods listed, have you experienced:	*19–24 mo. ago*	*13–18 mo. ago*	*7–12 mo. ago*	*0–6 mo. ago*	*Your Adjust. Score*
1. an illness or injury which:					
(a) kept you in bed a week or more, or took you to the hospital?	___	___	___	___	___
(b) was less serious than described above?	___	___	___	___	___
2. a major change in eating habits?	___	___	___	___	___
3. a major change in sleeping habits?	___	___	___	___	___
4. a change in your usual type and/or amount of recreation?	___	___	___	___	___
5. major dental work?	___	___	___	___	___

B. WORK

	19–24 mo. ago	*13–18 mo. ago*	*7–12 mo. ago*	*0–6 mo. ago*	*Your Adjust. Score*
6. changed to a new type of work?	___	___	___	___	___
7. changed your work hours or conditions?	___	___	___	___	___
8. had a change in your responsibilities at work:					
(a) more responsibilities?	___	___	___	___	___
(b) less responsibilities?	___	___	___	___	___
(c) promotion?	___	___	___	___	___
(d) demotion?	___	___	___	___	___
(e) transfer?	___	___	___	___	___
9. experienced trouble at work:					
(a) with your boss?	___	___	___	___	___
(b) with co-workers?	___	___	___	___	___
(c) with persons under your supervision?	___	___	___	___	___
(d) other work troubles?	___	___	___	___	___

Within the time periods listed, have you:	*19–24 mo. ago*	*13–18 mo. ago*	*7–12 mo. ago*	*0–6 mo. ago*	*Your Adjust. Score*
10. experienced a major business readjustment?	——	——	——	——	——
11. retired?	——	——	——	——	——
12. experienced being:					
(a) fired from work?	——	——	——	——	——
(b) laid off from work?	——	——	——	——	——
13. taken courses by mail or studied at home to help you in your work?	——	——	——	——	——

C. HOME AND FAMILY

Within the time periods listed, have you experienced:

	19–24 mo. ago	*13–18 mo. ago*	*7–12 mo. ago*	*0–6 mo. ago*	*Your Adjust. Score*
14. a change in residence:					
(a) a move within the same town or city?	——	——	——	——	——
(b) a move to a different town, city or state?	——	——	——	——	——
15. a change in family "get-togethers"?	——	——	——	——	——
16. a major change in the health or behavior of a family member (illnesses, accidents, drug or disciplinary problems, etc.)?	——	——	——	——	——
17. major change in your living conditions (home improvements or a decline in your home or neighborhood)?	——	——	——	——	——
18. the death of a spouse?	——	——	——	——	——
19. the death of a:					
(a) child?	——	——	——	——	——
(b) brother or sister?	——	——	——	——	——
(c) parent?	——	——	——	——	——
(d) other close family member?	——	——	——	——	——
20. the death of a close friend?	——	——	——	——	——
21. a change in the marital status of your parents:					
(a) divorce?	——	——	——	——	——
(b) remarriage?	——	——	——	——	——

Within the time periods listed, have you:	*19–24 mo. ago*	*13–18 mo. ago*	*7–12 mo. ago*	*0–6 mo. ago*	*Your Adjust. Score*
NOTE *(Questions 22–33 concern marriage. For persons never married, go to Item 34)*					
22. marriage?	———	———	———	———	———
23. a change in arguments with your spouse?	———	———	———	———	———
24. in-law problems?	———	———	———	———	———
25. a separation from spouse?					
27. a divorce?	———	———	———	———	———
28. a gain of a new family member:					
(a) birth of a child?	———	———	———	———	———
(b) adoption of a child?	———	———	———	———	———
(c) a relative moving in with you?	———	———	———	———	———
29. wife beginning or ceasing work outside the home?	———	———	———	———	———
30. wife becoming pregnant?	———	———	———	———	———
31. a child leaving home:					
(a) due to marriage?	———	———	———	———	———
(b) to attend college?	———	———	———	———	———
(c) for other reasons?	———	———	———	———	———
32. wife having a miscarriage or abortion?	———	———	———	———	
33. birth of a grandchild?	———	———	———	———	———

D. PERSONAL AND SOCIAL

Within the time periods listed, have you experienced:

	19–24 mo. ago	*13–18 mo. ago*	*7–12 mo. ago*	*0–6 mo. ago*	*Your Adjust. Score*
34. a major personal achievement?	———	———	———	———	———
35. a change in your personal habits (your dress, friends, life-style, etc.)?	———	———	———	———	———
36. sexual difficulties?	———	———	———	———	———
37. beginning or ceasing school or college?	———	———	———	———	———
38. a change of school or college?	———	———	———	———	———
39. a vacation?	———	———	———	———	———
40. a change in your religious beliefs?	———	———	———	———	———
41. a change in your social activities (clubs, movies, visiting)?	———	———	———	———	———
42. a minor violation of the law?	———	———	———	———	———

Within the time periods listed, have you:	*19–24* *mo. ago*	*13–18* *mo. ago*	*7–12* *mo. ago*	*0–6* *mo. ago*	*Your Adjust.* *Score*
43. legal troubles resulting in your being held in jail?	——	——	——	——	——
44. a change in your political beliefs?	——	——	——	——	——
45. a new, close, personal relationship?	——	——	——	——	——
46. an engagement to marry?	——	——	——	——	——
47. a "falling out" of a close personal relationship?	——	——	——	——	——
48. girlfriend (or boyfriend) problems?	——	——	——	——	——
49. a loss or damage of personal property?	——	——	——	——	——
50. an accident?	——	——	——	——	——
51. a major decision regarding your immediate future?	——	——	——	——	——

E. FINANCIAL
Within the time periods listed, have you:

52. taken on a moderate purchase, such as a T.V., car, freezer, etc.?	——	——	——	——	——
53. taken on a major purchase or a mortgage loan, such as a home, business, property, etc.?	——	——	——	——	——
54. experienced a foreclosure on a mortgage or loan?	——	——	——	——	——
55. experienced a major change in finances:					
(a) increased income?	——	——	——	——	——
(b) decreased income?	——	——	——	——	——
(c) credit rating difficulties?	——	——	——	——	——

Six-month LCU totals	——	——	——	——	——
Six-month SLCU totals	——	——	——	——	——

INSTRUCTIONS FOR SCORING YOUR ADJUSTMENT TO YOUR RECENT LIFE CHANGE

Persons adapt to their recent lefe changes in different ways. Some people find the adjustment to a residential move, for example, to be enormous, while others find very little life adjustment necessary. You are now requested to "score" each of the recent life changes that you marked with an "X" as to the amount of adjustment you needed to handle the event.

Your scores can range from 1 to 100 "points." If, for example, you experienced a recent residential move but felt it required very little life adjustment, you would choose a low number and place it in the blank to the right of the question's boxes. On the other hand, if you recently changed residence and felt it required a near maximal life adjustment, you would place a high number, toward 100, in the blank to the right of the question's boxes. For intermediate life adjustment scores you would choose intermediate numbers between 1 and 100.

Please go back through your questionnaire and for each recent life change you indicated with an "X," choose your personal life change adjustment score (between 1 and 100) which reflects what you saw to be the amount of life adjustment necessary to cope with or handle the event. Use both your estimates of the intensity of the life change and its duration to arrive at your scores.

From Rahe, R.H. Epidemiological Studies of Life Change and Illness. *The International Journal of Psychiatry in Medicine*, 6 (1/2), 133–146. © 1976,Bolywood Publishing Co., Inc.

CHAPTER
3 Transcultural Considerations in Assessment

Purpose: This chapter discusses the characteristics of culture, the dominant value orientation of various groups in North America, the cultural dimensions of health care, and the ways in which cultural practices affect health, illness, self care, and treatment measures. At the end of this unit, you should have increased sensitivity to the cultural dimensions of health care, and be able to perform a cultural assessment.

Reading Assignment: Jarvis, *Physical Examination and Health Assessment*, 2nd ed., Chapter 3, pp. 45–57; Chapter 5, pp. 95–96

Glossary: Study the following terms after reading the corresponding chapter in the text. You should be able to cover the definition on the right and define the term out loud.

Culture shock .... state of disorientation to a different cultural group because of its sudden strangeness, unfamiliarity, and incompatibility to person's perceptions and expectations

Folk healer .... lay healer in the person's culture apart from the biomedical/ scientific health care system

Lineal relationships .... ties with others by virtue of heredity and kinship

Religion .... an organized system of beliefs concerning the cause, nature, and purpose of the universe, especially a belief in God or gods

Spirituality .... each person's personal effort to find purpose and meaning in life

Subculture .... fairly large aggregates of people who have shared characteristics that are not common to all members of the culture

Yin/yang theory .... health exists when all aspects of the person are in perfect balance;

STUDY GUIDE

After completing the reading assignment, you should be able to answer the following questions in the spaces provided.

1. List the 4 basic characteristics of culture.

2. Define the term *dominant value orientation* and state what this represents in the United States.

3. List 3 major ways that people can perceive the time dimension, and give examples of cultural groups who hold each focus.

4. List and define 3 ways in which people's relationships with others may be categorized.

5. List 6 categories of families.

6. List and define 3 major theories in which people view the causes of illness.

7. Define the *yin/yang theory* of health and illness and relate this to different types of foods.

8. Define the *hot/cold theory* of health and illness, and relate this to different types of foods and illnesses.

9. List at least 5 names for various folk healers including the culture they represent.

10. Define the term *culture-bound syndrome*, and give examples from the black, Hispanic, Native American, and white cultures.

11. Give an example of a genetic trait or disorder commonly associated with the following populations or ethnic groups:

African_____

Ashkenazi Jews_____

Amish_____

Mediterraneans (Italians, Greeks) _____

REVIEW QUESTIONS

This test is for you and is intended to check your own mastery of the content. Answers are provided in Appendix A.

1. C.D. is a Lieutenant in the Navy. When considering culture as part of the assessment of this for this individual, the most obvious subculture is that of:
   a) sex
   b) occupation
   c) ethnicity
   d) health-related characteristics.

2. E. A. has brought M., age 5, to the clinic for a periodic health screening. Interview reveals that E. A. is married to M.'s father, but is not the child's biological mother. The three live together. This is an example of a:
   a) nuclear family.
   b) extended family.
   c) blended family.
   d) single family.

3. Religion is best described as:

   a)   an organized system of beliefs concerning the cause, nature, and purpose of the universe.

   b)   a unique life experience and personal effort to find purpose and meaning in life.

   c)   affiliation with one of the 1200 recognized religions in the United States

   d)   the following of established rituals, especially in conjunction with health seeking behaviors.

4. Belief regarding causes of illness are part of a cultures' view of health and illness. All of the theories listed below are discussed in the text except:

   a)   the biomedical theory.

   b)   the naturalistic theory.

   c)   the bio-psycho-social disorder theory.

   d)   the magico-religious theory.

5. Select the least accurate description of pain.

   a)   The manifestation and management of pain are embedded in a cultural context.

   b)   Pain is a universal phenomena, therefore its expression is also universal.

   c)   Pain is a highly personal experience, depending on cultural learning.

   d)   The term *pain* is derived from the Greek word for penalty.

6. B. D. has been diagnosed in-utero with spina bifida. This is an example of a(n):

   a)   disorder associated with a genetic trait.

   b)   culture-bound syndrome.

   c)   environmentally caused disorder.

   d)   disorder caused by nontraditional intervention during pregnancy.

SKILLS LABORATORY/ CLINICAL SETTING

You are now ready for the clinical component of the transcultural chapter. The purpose of the clinical component is to collect data for a cultural assessment on a peer in the skills laboratory or on a client in the clinical setting. Although you may not have been assigned chapters on the health history as yet, the questions in the cultural assessment tool are clearly defined and should pose no problem. The very best experience would be for you to pair up with a peer from a cultural group different from your own. If this is not possible, you still will gain insight and sensitivity into the cultural dimensions of health, and will gain mastery of the assessment tool.

Cultural Assessment

Brief History of the Cultural Group With Which the Person Identifies

(Record responses below)

- With what cultural group(s) do you affiliate (e.g., Hispanic, Polish, Navajo, or combination)? To what degree do you identify with the cultural group (e.g., "we" concept of solidarity or a fringe member)?
- What is your reported racial affiliation (e.g., black, Native American, Asian, and so on)?
- Where were you born?
- Where have you lived (country, city) and when (during what years)? Note: If a recent relocation to the United States, knowledge of prevalent diseases in country of origin may be helpful.

Values Orientation

- What are your attitudes, values, and beliefs about birth, death, health, illness, health care providers?
- How do you view work, leisure, education?
- How do you perceive change?

Cultural Sanctions and Restrictions

- How does your cultural group regard expression of emotion and feelings, spirituality, and religious beliefs? How are dying, death, and grieving expressed in a culturally appropriate manner?
- How is modesty expressed by men and women? Are there culturally defined expectations about male-female relationships, including the health care relationship?
- Do you have any restrictions related to sexuality, exposure of body parts, certain types of surgery (e.g., amputation, vasectomy, hysterectomy)?
- Are there any restrictions against discussion of dead relatives or fears related to the unknown?

Communication

- What language do you speak at home? What other languages do you speak or read? In what language would you prefer to communicate?
- Do you need an interpreter? If so, is there a relative or friend who would like to interpret? Is there anyone whom you would prefer did not interpret (e.g., member of the opposite sex, a person younger/older than you, member of a rival tribe or nation)?
- How do you feel about health care providers who are not of the same cultural background (e.g., black, middle-class nurse and Hispanic of a different social class)? Do you prefer to receive care from a nurse or doctor of the same cultural background, gender, and/or age?

Health-Related Beliefs and Practices

- To what cause(s) do you attribute illness and disease (e.g., divine wrath, imbalance in hot/cold or yin/yang, punishment for moral transgressions, hex, soul loss)?
- What do you believe promotes health (eating certain foods, wearing amulates to bring good luck, exercise, prayer, rituals to ancestors, saints, or intermediate deities)?
- What is your religious affiliation (e.g., Judaism, Islam, Pentecostalism, West African voodooism, Seventh-Day Adventism, Catholicism, Mormonism)?
- Do you rely on cultural healers (e.g., curandero, shaman, spiritualist, priest, minister, monk)? Who determines when you are sick and you are healthy? Who determines the type of healer and treatment that should be sought?
- In what types of cultural healing practices do you engage (use of herbal remedies, potions, massage, wearing of talismans or charms to discourage evil spirits, healing rituals, incantations, prayers)?
- How are biomedical/scientific health care providers perceived? How do you and your family perceive nurses or physicians? What are the expectations of nurses and nursing care?
- What is appropriate "sick role" behavior? Who determines what symptoms constitute disease/illness? Who decides when you are no longer sick? Who cares for you at home?
- How does your cultural group view mental disorders? Are there differences in acceptable behaviors for physical versus psychological illnesses?

Nutrition

- What is the meaning of food and eating to you? With whom do you usually eat? What types of foods are eaten? What do you define as food? What do you believe composes a "healthy" versus and "unhealthy"diet?
- How are foods prepared at home (type of food preparation, cooking oil(s) used, length of time foods are cooked, especially vegetables, amount and type of seasoning added to various foods during preparation)?

- Do religious beliefs and practices influence your diet (e.g., amount, type, preparation or delineation of acceptable food combinations, such as kosher diets)? Do you abstain from certain foods at regular intervals, on specific dates determined by the religious calendar, or at other times?

- If your religion mandates or encourages fasting, what does the term "fast" mean (e.g., refraining from certain types or quantities of foods, eating only during certain times of the day)? For what period of time are you expected to fast?

- During fasting, do you refrain from liquids/beverages? Does your religion allow exemption from fasting during illness? If so, do you believe that an exemption applies to you?

(Record responses below)

Socioeconomic Considerations

- Who composes your social network (family, peers, and cultural healers)? How do they influence your health or illness status?
- How do members of your social support network define caring (e.g., being continuously present, doing things for you, looking after your family)? What are the roles of various family members during health and illness?
- How does your family participate in the nursing care (e.g., bathing, feeding, touching, being present)?
- Does the cultural family structure influence your response to health or illness (e.g., beliefs, strenghts, weaknesses, and social class)? Is there a key family member whose role is significant in health-related decisions (e.g., grandmother in many black families, eldest adult son in Asian families)?
- Who is the principal wage earner in your family? What is the total annual income? (Note: This is a potentially sensitive question that should be asked only if necessary.) Is there more than one wage earner? Are there other sources of financial support (extended family, investments)?
- What impact does economic status have on lifestyle, place of residence, living conditions, ability to obtain health care, discharge planning?

Organizations Providing Cultural Support

- What influence do ethnic/cultural organizations have on your receiving health care (e.g., Organizations of Migrant Workers, National Association for the Advancement of Colored People (NAACP), Black Political Caucus, curches, schools, Urban League, community-based health care programs and clinics).

Educational Background

- What is your highest educational level obtained?
- Can you read and write English, or is another language preferred? If English is the second language, are materials available in the primary language?
- What learning style is most comfortable/familiar? Do you prefer to learn through written materials, oral explanation, or demonstration?

Religious Affiliation

- What is the role of religious beliefs and practices during health and illness?
- Are there healing rituals or practices that you believe can promote wellbeing or hasten recovery from illness? If so, who performs these?
- What is the role of significant religious representatives during health and illness? Are there recognized healers (e.g., Islamic imams, Christian Scientist practitioners or nurses, Catholic priests, Mormon elders, Buddhist monks)?

Spiritual Considerations

- Does the person have religious objects in the environment?
- Does the person wear outer- or undergarments having religious significance?
- Are get-well greeting cards religious in nature or from a religious represenative?
- Does the person appear to pray at certain times of the day or before meals?
- Does the person make special dietary requests (e.g., Kosher diet; vegetarian diet; diet free from caffeine, pork, shellfish, or other specific food items)?
- Does the person read religious magazines or books?
- Does the person mention God (Allah, Buddha, Yahweh, or a synonym), prayer, faith, or other religious topics?
- Is a request made for a visit by a member of the clergy or other religious representative?
- Is there an expression of anxiety or fear about pain, suffering, death?
- Does the person prefer to interact with others or to remain alone?

Data for spiritual considerations from Andrews MM, Hanson PA: Religion, culture, and nursing. In Boyle JS, Andrews MM (Eds). Transcultural Concepts in Nursing Care, 2nd ed. Philadelphia, J.B. Lippincott Company, 1995.

CHAPTER 4

The Interview

Purpose: This chapter discusses the process of communication; presents the techniques of interviewing including open-ended vs. closed questions, the 9 types of examiner responses, the 10 "traps" of interviewing, and nonverbal skills; and considers variations in technique that are necessary for clients of different ages, for those with special needs, and for culturally diverse clients.

Reading Assignment: Jarvis, *Physical Examination and Health Assessment*, 2nd ed., Chapter 4, pp. 59-77

_____

Audio-Visual Assignment: _____

_____

Glossary: Study the following terms after reading the corresponding chapter in the text. You should be able to cover the definition on the right and define the term out loud.

Animism	imagining that inanimate objects (e.g., blood pressure cuff) come alive and have human characteristics
Avoidance language	the use of euphemisms to avoid reality or to hide feelings
Clarification	examiner's response used when the client's word choice is ambiguous or confusing
Closed questions	questions that ask for specific information; elicit a short, one or two word answer, a yes or no, or a forced choice
Confrontation	response in which examiner gives honest feedback about what he or she has seen or felt after observing a certain client action, feeling, or statement
Distancing	the use of impersonal speech to put space between the self and a threat
Empathy	viewing the world from the other person's inner frame of reference while remaining yourself; recognizing and accepting the other person's feelings without criticism
Ethnocentrism	the tendency to view your own way of life as the most desirable, acceptable, or best and to act in a superior manner to another culture's lifeways
Explanation	examiner's statements that inform the client; examiner shares factual and objective information

Facilitation .... examiner's response that encourages the client to say more, to continue with the story

Interpretation .... examiner's statement that is not based on direct observation, but is based on examiner's inference or conclusion; it links events, makes associations, or implies cause

Interview .... meeting between examiner and client with the goal of gathering a complete health history

Jargon .... using medical vocabulary with clients in an exclusionary and paternalistic way

Leading question .... a question that implies that one answer would be better than another

Nonverval communication .... message conveyed through posture, gestures, facial expression, eye contact, touch, and even when one places the chairs

Open-ended questions .... asks for longer narrative information; unbiased, leaves the person free to answer in any way

Reflection .... examiner response that echoes the client's words; repeats part of what client has just said

Summary .... final review of what examiner understands client has said; condenses facts and presents a survey of how the examiner perceives the health problem or need

Verbal communication .... messages sent through spoken words, vocalizations, tone of voice

STUDY GUIDE

After completing the reading assignment and the audio-visual assignment, you should be able to answer the following questions in the spaces provided.

1. List 8 items of information that should be communicated to the client concerning the terms or expectations of the interview.

2. Describe the points to consider in preparing the physical setting for the interview.

3. List the pros and cons of note-taking during the interview.

4. Contrast open-ended vs. closed questions and explain the purpose of each during the interview.

5. List the 9 types of examiner responses that could be used during the interview, and give a short example of each.

6. List the 10 traps of interviewing, and give a short example of each.

7. State at least 7 types of nonverbal behaviors that an interviewer could make.

8. State a useful phrase to use as a closing when ending the interview.

9. Discuss special considerations when interviewing the older adult.

10. Discuss ways you would modify your interviewing technique when working with a hearing-impaired person.

11. Formulate a response you would make to a client who has spoken to you in ways you interpret as sexually aggressive.

12. Discuss the ways that nonverval behavior may vary cross culturally.

13. List at least 5 points to consider when using an interpreter during an interview.

REVIEW QUESTIONS

This test is for you and is intended to check your own mastery of the content. Answers are provided in Appendix A.

1. The practitioner, entering the examining room to meet a client for the first time, states: "Hello, I'm M.M. and I'm here to gather some information from you and to perform your examination. This will take about 30 minutes. D.D. is a student working with me. If it's all right with you, she will remain during the examination." Which of the following must be added in order to cover all aspects of the interview contract?

   a) A statement regarding confidentiality, client costs, and the expectation of each person.
   b) The purpose of the interview and the role of the examiner.
   c) Time and place of the interview and a confidentiality statement.
   d) An explicit purpose of the interview and a description of the physical examination, including diagnostic studies.

2. Unconditional positive regard toward a client within a communication context is an example of:

   a) empathy.
   b) liking others.
   c) empathizing with the client.
   d) a nonverbal listening technique.

3. The nurse has come into a client's room to conduct an admission interview. Because the nurse is expecting a phone call, the nurse stands near the door during the interview. A more appropriate approach would be to:

   a) arrange to have someone page you so you can sit on the side of the bed.
   b) have someone answer the phone and sit facing the client.
   c) use this approach given the circumstances; it is correct.
   d) arrange for a time free of interruptions until the initial physical examination is complete.

4. Students frequently ask teachers "May I ask you a question?" This is an example of:

   a) an open-ended question.
   b) A direct question.
   c) a closed question
   d) a double barreled question.

5. During a client interview, the nurse recognizes the need to use interpretation. This verbal response:

   a)   is the same as clarification
   b)   is summary of a statement made by a client.
   c)   is used to focus on a particular aspect of what the client has just said.
   d)   is based on the interviewer's inference from the data that has been presented.

6. A good rule for an interviewer is to:

   a)   Stop the client each time something is said that is not understood.
   b)   Spend more time listening to the client than talking.
   c)   Consistently think of your next response so the client will know you understand him.
   d)   Use "why" questions to seek clarification of unusual symptoms or behavior.

7. During an interview, a client denies having any anxiety. The client frequently changes position in the chair and has little eye contact with the interviewer. The interviewer should:

   a)   use confrontation to bring the discrepancy between verbal and nonverbal behavior to the client's attention.
   b)   proceed with the interview. Client's usually are truthful with a health care practitioner.
   c)   make a mental note to discuss the behavior after the physical examination is completed.
   d)   proceed with the interview and exam as outlined on the agency assessment form. The client's behavior is appropriate for the circumstances.

8. Touch should be used during the interview:

   a)   only with clients from a Western culture.
   b)   as a way of establishing contact with the client and communicating empathy.
   c)   only with clients of the same sex.
   d)   only if the interviewer knows the person well.

9. Children are usually brought for health care by a parent. At what age should the interviewer begin to question the child regarding presenting symptoms?

   a)   5.
   b)   7.
   c)   9.
   d)   11.

10. Because of their developmental level, not all interviewing techniques can be used with adolescents. The two to be avoided are:

   a)   Facilitation and clarification.
   b)   Confrontation and explanation.
   c)   Empathy and interpretations.
   d)   Silence and reflection.

11. Knowledge of the use of personal space is helpful for the health care provider. Personal distance is generally considered to be:

   a)   0 to 1 1/2 feet
   b)   1 1/2 to 4 feet
   c)   4 to 12 feet
   d)   12 or more feet.

Note that the clinical component of this chapter is the gathering of the complete health history. The history forms are included in Chapter 5.

CHAPTER 5

The Complete Health History

Purpose: This chapter helps you to learn the elements of a complete health history, to interview a client to gather the data for a complete health history, to analyze the client data, and to record the history accurately.

Reading Assignment: Jarvis, *Physical Examination and Health Assessment*, 2nd ed., Chapter 5, pp. 80-97

STUDY GUIDE

After completing the reading assignment, you should be able to answer the following questions in the spaces provided.

1. State the purpose of the complete health history.

2. List and define the critical characteristics used to explore each symptom the client identifies.

3. Define the elements of the health history: reason for seeking care; present health state or present illness; past history, family history; review of systems; functional patterns of living.

4. Discuss the rationale for obtaining a family history.

5. Discuss the rationale for obtaining a systems review.

6. Describe the items included in a functional assessment.

7. Describe the additions/modifications you would make in environment, pacing and content when conducting a health history on an older adult.

REVIEW QUESTIONS

This test is for you and is intended to check your own mastery of the content. Answers are provided in Appendix A.

1. The practitioner reading a medical record sees the following notation: "Client states 'I have had a cold for about a week and now I am having difficulty breathing'." This is an example of:

   a) Past history.
   b) Review of systems.
   c) A functional assessment.
   d) Reason for seeking care.

2. A practitioner has reason to question the reliability of the information being provided by a client. One way to verify the reliability within the context of the interview is to:

   a) Rephrase the same questions later in the interview.
   b) Review the client's previous medical records.
   c) Call the person identified as emergency contact to verify data provided.
   d) Provide the client with a printed history to complete and then compare the data provided.

3. The statement "Reason for seeking care" has replaced the "Chief Complaint." This change is significant because:

   a) "Chief Complaint" is really a diagnostic statement.
   b) The newer term allows another individual to supply the necessary information.
   c) The newer term incorporates wellness needs.
   d) "Reason for seeking care" can incorporate the history of present illness.

4. During an initial interview, the examiner asks "Mrs. J., tell me what you do when your headaches occur." With this question, the examiner is seeking information about:

   a) The client's perception of the problem.
   b) Aggravating or relieving factors.
   c) The frequency of the problem.
   d) The severity of the problem.

5. K. M., who now has a seizure disorder, states that he had an auto accident at age 19. This information would be considered a past health history of:

   a) accidents and chronic illnesses.
   b) childhood illnesses and hospitalizations.
   c) current medication and serious illnesses
   d) accidents only.

6. A genogram is useful in showing information concisely. It is used specifically for:

   a) past history
   b) past health history, specifically hospitalizations.
   c) family history.
   d) the eight characteristics of presenting symptoms.

7. Select the best description of "review of systems" as part of the health history.

   a) The evaluation of the past and present health state of each body system.
   b) A documentation of the problem as described by the client.
   c) The recording of the objective findings of the practitioner.
   d) A statement that describes the overall health state of the client.

8. During an initial meeting with a new client, the practitioner interviews the client about the use of alcohol. This is part of a:

   a) functional assessment.
   b) nutritional assessment.
   c) health promotion assessment.
   d) family history assessment.

9. When taking a health history for a child, what information in addition to that for an adult, is usually obtained?

   a) Coping and stress management.
   b) A review of immunizations received.
   c) Environmental hazards.
   d) Hospitalization history.

10. Functional assessment measures how a person manages day-to-day activities. The impact of a disease on the daily activities of older adults is referred to as:

    a)   Interpersonal relationship assessment.
    b)   Instrumental activities of daily living.
    c)   Reason for seeking care.
    d)   Disease burden.

SKILLS LABORATORY/CLINICAL SETTING

You are now ready for the clinical component of the Interview and Health History chapters. The purpose of the clinical component is to practice conducting a complete health history on a peer in the skills laboratory and to achieve the following.

Clinical Objectives

1. Demonstrate knowledge of interviewing skills by: arranging a private, quiet, comfortable setting; introducing yourself and stating your goals for the interview; posing open-ended and direct questions appropriately; listening to the client in an attentive, nonjudgmental manner; choosing appropriate vocabulary that the client understands.

2. Demonstrate knowledge of the components of a health history by: recording the reason for seeking care in the person's own words; eliciting all the critical characteristics to describe the client's symptom(s); gathering pertinent data for the past history, family history, and systems review; identifying self-care behaviors and risk factors from the functional assessment.

3. Record the history data accurately and as a reflection of what the client believes the true health state to be.

Instructions

Work in pairs and obtain a complete health history from a peer. Although you already know each other as student colleagues, play your role straight as examiner or client for the best learning experience. Be aware that some of the history questions cover personal content. When you are acting as the client, you have the right to withhold an answer if you do not feel comfortable with the amount of material you will be asked to divulge. Your own rights to privacy must co-exist with the goals of the learning experience.

Familiarize yourself with the following history form and practice phrasing your questions ahead of time. Note that the language on this form is intended as a prompt for the examiner, and must be translated into clear and appropriate phrases for the client. As a beginning examiner, you will need to use one copy of the form as a worksheet during the actual interview, and use a fresh copy of the form for your rewritten formal record.

CHAPTER 6

Mental Status Assessment

Purpose: This chapter helps you learn the components of the mental status examination including assessing a person's appearance, behavior, cognitive functions, and thought processes and perceptions; to understand the rationale and methods of examination of mental status; and to record the assessment accurately.

Reading Assignment: Jarvis, *Physical Examination and Health Assessment*, 2nd ed., Chapter 6, pp. 100-124

Glossary: Study the following terms after completing the reading assignment. You should be able to cover the definition on the right and define the term out loud.

Abstract reasoning .... pondering a deeper meaning beyond the concrete and literal

Attention .... concentration, ability to focus on one specific thing

Consciousness .... being aware of one's own existence, feelings, and thoughts and being aware of the environment

Language .... using the voice to communicate one's thoughts and feelings

Memory .... ability to lay down and store experiences and perceptions for later recall

Mood .... prolonged display of a person's feelings

Orientation .... awareness of the objective world in relation to the self

Perceptions .... awareness of objects through any of the five senses

Thought content .... *what* the person thinks — specific ideas, beliefs, the use of words

Thought process .... the *way* a person thinks, the logical train of thought

STUDY GUIDE

After completing the reading assignment, you should be able to answer the following questions in the spaces provided.

   1. Define the term *mental disorder*.

   2. List 4 situations in which it would be necessary to perform a complete mental status examination.

   3. Explain 4 factors that could affect the client's response to the mental status examination, but have nothing to do with mental disorders.

   4. Distinguish *dysphonia* from *dysarthria*.

   5. Define *unilateral neglect*, and state the illness with which it is associated.

   6. State convenient ways to assess a person's recent memory within the context of the initial health history.

   7. Which mental function is the Four Unrelated Words Test intended to test?

8. List at least 3 questions you could ask a client that would screen for suicide ideation.

9. Describe the client response level of consciousness that would be graded as:

Lethargic or somnolent _____

Obtunded _____

Stupor or semi-coma_____

Coma _____

Delirium_____

10. State the symptoms and physical signs that are characteristic of alcohol withdrawal.

REVIEW QUESTIONS

This test is for you and is intended to check your own mastery of the content. Answers are provided in Appendix A.

1. Although a full mental status examination may not be required, the examiner must be aware of the four main headings of the assessment while performing the interview and physical examination. These headings are:

   a) mood, affect, consciousness and orientation.
   b) memory, attention, thought content and perceptions.
   c) language, orientation, attention and abstract reasoning.
   d) appearance, behavior, cognition and thought processes

2. Select the finding that most accurately describes the appearance of a client.

   a) Tense posture and restless activity. Clothing clean but of questionable appropriateness for season; client wearing Tee shirt and shorts in October.
   b) Oriented times 3. Affect appropriate for circumstances.
   c) Alert and responds to verbal stimuli. Tearful when diagnosis discussed.
   d) Laughing inappropriately, oriented times 3.

3. The ability to lay down new memories is part of the assessment of cognitive functions. One way to accomplish this is with:

   a) Noting whether the client completes a thought without wandering.
   b) A test of general knowledge.
   c) A description of past medical history.
   d) The four unrelated words test.

4. In order to accurately plan for discharge teaching, additional assessments may be required for the client with aphasia. This may be accomplished by asking the client to:

   a) remember four unrelated words 5 minutes after they have been first introduced to the client.
   b) name his or her grandchildren and their birthdays.
   c) make up and write a sentence.
   d) interpret a proverb.

5. During an interview with a client newly diagnosed with a seizure disorder the client states "I plan to be an airline pilot." If the client continues to have this as a career goal after teaching regarding seizure disorders has been provided, the practitioner might question the client's:

   a) thought processes.
   b) judgment.
   c) attention span.
   d) recent memory.

6. On a client's second day in an acute care hospital, the client complains to the nurse about the "bugs" on the bed. The bed is clean. This would be an example of altered:

   a) thought process.
   b) orientation.
   c) perception.
   d) higher intellectual function.

7. Client's with organic brain disease may learn to conceal actual or perceived deficits. One way to assess cognitive function and to detect dementia is with:

   a) The Proverb Interpretation Test.
   b) The Mini-Mental State Examination.
   c) The Four Unrelated Words Test.
   d) The Older Adult Behavioral Checklist.

8. The Behavioral Checklist, completed by a parent, is used to assess the mental status of:

   a) infants.
   b) children 1 to 5 years of age
   c) children ages 7 1o 11 of age.
   d) adolescents.

9. A major characteristic of dementia is:

   a) impairment of short- and long-term memory.
   b) hallucinations.
   c) sudden onset of symptoms.
   d) it is substance-induced.

Match column B to with column A

Column A -Definition		Column B - Type of mood and affect	
10. ___	Lack of emotional response	a)	Depression
11. ___	Loss of Identity	b)	Anxiety
12. ___	Excessive well-being	c)	Flat affect
13. ___	Apprehensive from the anticipation of a danger whose source is unknown	d)	Euphoria
14. ___	Annoyed, easily provoked	e)	Lability
15. ___	Loss of control	f)	Rage
16. ___	Sad, gloomy, dejected	g)	Irritability
17. ___	Rapid shift of emotions	h)	Fear
18. ___	Worried about known external danger	i)	Depersonalization

19. Write a narrative account of a mental status assessment with normal findings.

SKILLS LABORATORY/CLINICAL SETTING

You are now ready for the clinical component of the mental status examination. The purpose of the clinical component is to achieve beginning competency with the administration of the mental status examination, and with the supplemental "Mini-Mental State" examination.

Practice the steps of the full mental status examination on a peer or a client in the clinical setting, giving appropriate instructions as you proceed. Formulate your questions to pose to the client ahead of time. Record your findings using the regional write-up sheet that follows.

Next practice the steps of the Mini-Mental State examination, which is a simplified scored form of the cognitive functions found on the full mental status examination. It is used frequently in clinical and research settings.

NOTES

NOTES

Nutritional Assessment

Purpose: This chapter helps you to learn the components of nutritional assessment, including the measurement of indicators of dietary status and nutrition-related health status of individuals; to identify the possible occurrence, nature, and extent of impaired nutritional status (ranging from deficiency to toxicity), and to record the assessment accurately.

Reading Assignment: Jarvis, *Physical Examination and Health Assessment*, 2nd ed., Chapter 7, pp. 125-156

Glossary: Study the following terms after completing the reading assignment. You should be able to cover the definition on the right and define the term out loud.

Acromion process .... the outer tip of the scapula that is used as an anatomic landmark in arm anthropometric measurements (e.g., midarm circumference, triceps skinfold)

Albumin   .... a serum protein produced by the liver and used as an indicator of nutritional status

Android obesity .... excess body fat that is placed predominantly within the abdomen and upper body as opposed to the hips and thighs

Anergy   .... a less-than-expected or absent immune reaction in response to the injection of antigens within the skin

Anthropometry .... measurement of the body, e.g., height weight, circumferences, skinfold thickness

Arm muscle area (AMA).......... an indicator of total body muscle calculated from the triceps skinfold thickness and midarm circumference

Body mass index .... Weight in kilograms divided by height in meters squared (W/H^2); value of 27 or > is indicative of obesity

Creatinine .... end product of creatine metabolism; 24 hour urinary creatinine excretion is used as an index of body muscle mass

Creatinine-height index (CHI) . index or ratio sometimes used to assess body protein status

Gynoid obesity .... excess body fat that is placed predominantly within the hips and thighs

Kwashiorkor .... primarily a protein deficiency characterized by edema, growth failure, and muscle wasting

Malnutrition .... may mean any nutrition disorder but usually refers to long-term nutritional inadequacies or excesses

Marasmic kwashiorkor .... combination of chronic energy deficit and chronic or acute protein deficiency

Marasmus .... results from energy and protein deficiency presenting with significant loss of body weight, skeletal muscle, and adipose tissue mass, but with serum protein concentrations relatively intact

Negative nitrogen balance .... condition in which nitrogen loss from the body exceeds nitrogen intake; often occurs with chronic illness, trauma, burns, recovery from major surgery

Nitrogen balance .... condition in which nitrogen losses from the body are equal to nitrogen intake; the expected state of the healthy adult

Nomogram .... graphic device with several vertical scales allowing calculation of certain values

Nutritional monitoring .... assessment of dietary or nutritional status at intermittent times with the aim of detecting changes in the dietary or nutritional status of a population

Obesity .... excessive accumulation of body fat; usually defined as 20% above desirable weight

Overnutrition .... condition resulting from the excessive intake of foods in general or particular food components

Protein-calorie malnutrition (PCM) .... inadequate consumption of protein and energy resulting in a gradual body wasting and increased susceptibility to infection

Recommended daily allowance .... levels of intake of essential nutrients considered to be adequate to meet the nutritional needs of practically all healthy persons

Resting energy expenditure (REE) .... the resting metabolic rate or the energy expenditure in the awake, resting, postabsorptive subject

Rickets .... condition especially found in infants and children characterized by malformed bones, delayed fontanel closure, and muscle pain, due to a deficiency of vitamin D

Scurvy .... an ascorbic acid (vitamin C) deficiency disease characterized by anemia, spongy and bleeding gums, and capillary hemorrhages

Serum proteins .... proteins present in serum that are indicators of the body's visceral protein status (e.g., albumin)

Skinfold thickness ....double fold of skin and underlying subcutaneous tissue that is measured with skinfold calipers at various body sites

Somatic protein.....................................protein contained in the body's skeletal muscles

Transferrin ....form in which iron is transported within the blood

Ulna ....larger inner bone of the forearm that is used as an anatomic landmark in arm anthropometry

Undernutrition ....condition resulting from the inadequate intake of food in general or particular food components

Visceral protein ....protein found in body's organs, in the serum, and in blood cells

Waist-to-hip ratio (WHR) ....waist or abdominal circumference divided by the hip or gluteal circumference; method for assessing fat distribution

STUDY GUIDE

After completing the reading assignment, you should be able to answer the following questions in the spaces provided.

1. Define *nutritional status.*

2. Describe the unique nutritional needs for various developmental periods throughout the life cycle.

3. Describe the role cultural heritage and values may play in an individual's nutritional intake.

4. State 3 purposes of a nutritional assessment.

5. List and describe 5 factors that identify the need for a comprehensive nutritional assessment for an individual.

6. Describe 4 sources of error that may occur when using the 24 hour diet recall.

7. Explain the clinical changes associated with each type of malnutrition:

Obesity _____

Marasmus _____

Kwashiorkor _____

Marasmus/Kwashiorkor mix _____

REVIEW QUESTIONS

This test is for you and is intended to check your own mastery of the content. Answers are provided in Appendix A.

1. The balance between nutrient intake and nutrient requirements is described as:

   a)   undernutrition
   b)   malnutrition.
   c)   nutritional status
   d)   overnutrition.

2. To support the synthesis of maternal and fetal tissue during pregnancy a weight gain of __pounds is recommended.

   a)   25 to 35 pounds
   b)   28 to 40 pounds
   c)   15 to 25 pounds
   d)   recommendation depends on BMI of mother at the start of the pregnancy

3. Which of the following are normal, expected, changes with aging?

   a)   moderate obesity
   b)   increase in muscle mass
   c)   decrease in height
   d)   decrease in arm span

4. Which of the following data would be obtained as part of a nutritional screening:

   a)   temperature, pulse, and respiration
   b)   blood pressure and genogram
   c)   height, weight, and part of the health history
   d)   past medical history

5. Current dietary guidelines recommend that complex carbohydrates comprise__% of total calorie intake:

   a) 30
   b) 40
   c) 50
   d) 75

6. The 24-hour recall of dietary intake:

   a) is an anthropometric measure of calories consumed.
   b) may be a questionnaire regarding everything eaten within the last 24 hours.
   c) is the same as a food frequency questionnaire.
   d) is a form of food diary.

7. The nutritional needs of a client with trauma or surgery:

   a) are met by body reserves in obese individuals.
   b) may be two to three times greater than normal.
   c) can be met with intravenous fluids, supplemented with vitamins and electrolytes.
   d) may increase 25% over usual intake.

8. Mary, a 15-year-old teen, has come for a school physical. During the interview, the examiner is told that menarche has not occurred. An explanation to be explored is:

   a) nutritional deficiency.
   b) alcohol intake.
   c) smoking history.
   d) possible elevated blood sugar.

9. Older adults are at risk for alteration in nutritional status. From the individuals described below, select the individual(s) who appear(s) least at risk.

   a) A 60-year-old widow who lives alone
   b) A 65-year-old widower who visits a senior center with a meal program, 5 days a week
   c) A 70 year old with poor dentition who lives with a son
   d) A 73-year-old couple with low income and no transportation

10. Body weight as a percentage of ideal body weight is calculated to assess for malnutrition. Severe malnutrition is:

    a) 80 to 90 percent of ideal weight.
    b) 70 to 80 percent of ideal weight.
    c) less than 70 percent of ideal body weight.
    d) 120 percent of ideal body weight.

11. The examiner is completing an initial assessment for a client being admitted to a long term care facility. The client is unable to stand for a measurement of height. In order to obtain this important anthropometric information the examiner may:

    a) ask the client how tall he or she is.
    b) obtain the information from the medical record of the transferring agency.
    c) measure arm span.
    d) obtain a mid-upper arm muscle circumference to estimate skeletal muscle reserve.

12. An anergy panel has been ordered for a client. This test is done to:

    a) obtain an indirect measure of total lymphocyte count.
    b) determine the need for adult immunization.
    c) assess for exposure to tuberculosis.
    d) assess for immunoincompetence.

SKILLS LABORATORY/ CLINICAL SETTING

You are now ready for the clinical component of the nutritional assessment. The purpose of the clinical component is to practice the steps of the assessment on a peer in the skills laboratory and to achieve the following.

Clinical Objectives

1. Identify persons at risk for developing malnutrition.

2. Develop an appreciation for cultural influences on nutritional status.

3. Use anthromometric measures and laboratory data to assess the nutritional status of an individual.

4. Use nutritional assessment in the provision of health care.

5. Record the assessment findings accurately.

Instructions

Gather nutritional assessment forms and anthropometric equipment. Practice the steps of the *Screening Nutritional Assessment Form* on a peer in the skills laboratory. This will familiarize you with the appropirate history questions and give you practice computing the derived weight measures. Likely you will not have access to a peer's serum laboratory data, however, the history and physical exam data will give you all the data you need to make a clinical judgment on a well adult. Record your findings using one of the Assessment Forms that follow.

Next, practice the steps of the *Comprehensive Nutritional Assessment Form* on a peer in the skills laboratory or on a client in the clinical setting. This will give you practice with a more detailed history, collecting food intake measures, physical examination signs, and performing anthropometric measures.

CHAPTER 8

Assessment Techniques and Approach to the Clinical Setting

Purpose: This chapter helps you to learn the assessment techniques of inspection, palpation, percussion, auscultation; to learn the items of equipment needed for a complete physical examination; and to consider age-specific modifications you would make for the examination of individuals throughout the life cycle.

Reading Assignment: Jarvis, *Physical Examination and Health Assessment*, 2nd ed., Chapter 8, pp. 161-173

Glossary: Study the following terms after completing the reading assignment. You should be able to cover the definition on the right and define the term out loud.

Amplitude	(or intensity), how loud or soft a sound is
Duration	the length of time a note lingers
Ophthalmoscope	instrument that illuminates the internal eye structures, enabling the examiner to look through the pupil at the fundus (background) of the eye
Otoscope	instrument that illuminates the ear canal, enabling the examiner to look at the ear canal and tympanic membrane
Pitch	(or frequency), the number of vibrations (or cycles) per second of a note
Quality	(or timbre), a subjective difference in a sound due to the sound's distinctive overtones

STUDY GUIDE

After completing the reading assignment, you should be able to answer the following questions in the spaces provided.

1. Define and describe the technique of the 4 physical examination skills:

    Inspection _____

    Palpation _____

    Percussion _____

    Auscultation _____

2. Define the characteristics of the following percussion notes:

	Pitch	Amplitude	Quality	Duration
Resonance				
Hyperresonance				
Tympany				
Dull				
Flat				

3. Differentiate direct percussion from indirect percussion.

4. Relate the parts of the hands to palpation techniques used in assessment.

5. Differentiate between light, deep, and bimanual palpation.

6. List the two endpieces of the stethoscope and the conditions for which each is best suited.

7. Describe the environmental conditions to consider in preparing the examination setting.

8. List the 20 basic items of equipment necessary to conduct a complete physical examination on an adult.

9. Describe your own preparation as you encounter the client for examination: your own dress, your demeanor, safety/universal precautions, sequence of examination steps, instructions to client.

10. What age specific considerations would you make for the examination of the:

Infant _____

Toddler _____

Preschooler _____

School-aged child _____

Adolescent _____

Older adult _____

Acutely ill person _____

REVIEW QUESTIONS

This test is for you and is intended to check your own mastery of the content. Answers are provided in Appendix A.

1. Various parts of the hands are used during palpation. The part of the hand used for the assessment of vibration is (are) the:

   a)   fingertips.
   b)   index finger and thumb in opposition.
   c)   dorsa of the hand.
   d)   ulnar surface of the hand.

2. When performing indirect percussion, the stationary finger is struck:

   a)   at the ulnar surface.
   b)   at the middle joint.
   c)   at the distal interphalangeal joint.
   d)   where ever it is in contact with the skin.

3. The best description of the pitch of a sound wave obtained by percussion is:

   a)   the intensity of the sound.
   b)   the number of vibrations per second.
   c)   the length of time the note lingers.
   d)   the overtones of the note.

4. The bell of the stethoscope:

   a)   is used for soft, low-pitched sounds.
   b)   is used for high-pitched sounds.
   c)   is held firmly against the skin.
   d)   magnifies sound.

5. The ophthalmoscope has five apertures. Which aperture would be used to assess the eyes of a client with undilated pupils?

   a)   grid
   b)   slit
   c)   small
   d)   large

6. At the conclusion of the examination, the examiner should:

   a)   document findings before leaving the examining room.
   b)   have findings confirmed by another practitioner.
   c)   relate objective findings to the subjective findings for accuracy.
   d)   summarize findings.

7. When the practitioner enters the examining room the infant client is asleep. The practitioner would best start the exam with:

   a)   height and weight.
   b)   blood pressure.
   c)   heart, lung, and abdomen.
   d)   temperature.

8. The sequence of an examination changes from beginning with the thorax to that of head to toe with what age child?

   a)   the infant
   b)   the preschool child
   c)   the school-age child
   d)   the adolescent

SKILLS LABORATORY/CLINICAL SETTING

Note that the clinical component of this chapter is combined with Chapter 9. Instructions and regional write-up forms are listed at the end of Chapter 9.

CHAPTER 9

General Survey, Measurement, Vital Signs

Purpose: This chapter helps you to learn the method of gathering data for a general survey on a client; and the techniques for measuring height, weight, and vital signs.

Reading Assignment: Jarvis, *Physical Examination and Health Assessment*, 2nd ed., Chapter 9, pp. 176-211

Glossary: Study the following terms after completing the reading assignment. You should be able to cover the definition on the right and define the term out loud.

Auscultatory gap .... a brief time period when Korotkoff's sounds disappear during auscultation of B/P; usually significant of hypertension

Bradycardia .... heart rate < 60 beats per minute in the adult

Sphygmomanometer .... instrument for measuring arterial blood pressure

Stroke volume .... amount of blood pumped out of the heart with each heartbeat

Tachycardia .... heart rate of > 100 beats per minute in the adult

STUDY GUIDE

After completing the reading assignment, you should be able to answer the following questions in the spaces provided.

1. List the significant information considered in each of the four areas of a general survey—physical appearance, body structure, mobility, and behavior.

2. Describe the normal posture and body build.

3. Note aspects of normal gait.

4. Describe the clinical appearance of the following variations in stature:

Hypopituitary dwarfism _____

Gigantism _____

Acromegaly _____

Achrondroplastic dwarfism _____

Marfan's syndrome _____

Endogenous obesity (Cushing's syndrome) _____

Anorexia nervosa _____

5. State the normal weight range for a male, 5'10" tall, medium frame _____; for a female 5'4" tall, medium frame _____.

6. For serial weight measurements, what time of day would you instruct the person to have the weight measured? _____

7. Describe the technique for mesuring head circumference and chest circumference on an infant.

8. What changes in height and in weight distribution would you expect for an adult in their 70s and 80s.

9. Describe the tympanic membrane thermometer, and compare its use to other forms of temperature measurement.

10. Describe 4 qualities to consider when assessing the pulse.

11. Relate the qualities of normal respirations to the appropriate approach to counting them.

12. Define and describe the relationships among the terms *blood pressure, systolic pressure, diastolic pressure*, and *pulse pressure*.

13. List factors that affect blood pressure.

14. Relate the use of an improper size blood pressure cuff to the possible findings that may be obtained.

15. Explain the significance of Phase I, Phase IV, and Phase V Korotkoff sounds during B/P measurement.

16. Given an apparently healthy, 20-year-old adult, state the expected range for oral temperature, pulse, respirations, and blood pressure.

17. List the parameters of High Normal blood pressure, Stage 1 or Mild hypertension, and Stage 2 or Moderate hypertension.

REVIEW QUESTIONS

This test is for you and is intended to check your own mastery of the content. Answers are provided in Appendix A.

1. The four areas to consider during the general survey are:

   a)   ethnicity, sex, age, and socioeconomic status.
   b)   physical appearance, sex, ethnicity, and affect.
   c)   dress, affect, nonverbal behavior, and mobility.
   d)   physical appearance, body structure, mobility, and behavior.

2. During the general survey part of the exam, gait is assessed. When walking, the base is usually:

   a)   varied, depending upon the height of the client.
   b)   equal to the length of the arm.
   c)   as wide as the shoulder width.
   d)   1/2 of the height of the client.

3. A child, 18 months in age, is brought in for a health screening visit. To asses the height of the child:

   a)   use a tape measure .
   b)   use a horizontal measuring board.
   c)   have the child stand on the upright scale.
   d)   measure arm span to estimate height.

4. B. D. was delivered by cesarean section at 38 weeks of gestation because of fetal distress. She weighed 6 lbs., 4 oz. This weight :

   a)   is appropriate for gestational age.
   b)   is small for gestational age.
   c)   is large for gestational age.
   d)   cannot be determined from available data.

5. During the 8th and 9th decade of life, physical changes occur. Height and weight:

   a)   both increase.
   b)   weight increases, height decreases.
   c)   both decrease.
   d)   remain the same as during the 70s

6. During an initial home visit, the client's temperature is noted to be 97.4° F. This temperature:

   a)   cannot be evaluated without a knowledge of the client's age.
   b)   is below normal. The client should be assessed for possible hypothermia.
   c)   should be retaken by the rectal route, since this best reflects core body temperature.
   d)   should be reevaluated at the next visit before a decision is made.

7. Select the best description of an accurate assessment of a client's pulse.

   a)   count for 15 seconds if pulse is regular
   b)   begin counting with zero, count for 30 seconds
   c)   count for 30 seconds and multiply by 2
   d)   count for one full minute, begin counting with zero

8. After assessing the client's pulse, the practitioner determines it to be "normal" This would be recorded as:

   a)   3+
   b)   2+
   c)   1+
   d)   0

9. Select the best description of an accurate assessment of a client's respirations.

   a) count for a full minute before taking the pulse
   b) count for 15 seconds and multiply by 4
   c) count after informing the client where you are in the assessment process
   d) count for 30 seconds following pulse assessment

10. Pulse pressure is:

   a) the difference between the systolic and diastolic pressure.
   b) a reflection of the viscosity of the blood.
   c) another way to express the systolic pressure.
   d) a measure of vasoconstriction.

11. The examiner is going to assess for coarctation of the aorta. In an individual with coarctation the thigh pressure would be:

   a) higher than in the arm
   b) equal to that in the arm.
   c) there is no constant relationship. Findings are highly individual.
   d) lower than in the arm.

SKILLS LABORATORY/CLINICAL SETTING

You are now ready for the clinical component of Chapters 8 and 9. The purpose of the clinical component is to observe and describe the regional examination on a peer in the skills laboratory and to achieve the following.

Clinical Objectives

1. Observe and describe the significant characteristics of a general survey.

2. Measure height and weight and determine if findings are within normal range.

3. Gather vital signs data.

4. Record the physical examination findings accurately.

Instructions

Set up your section of the skills laboratory for a complete physical examination, attending to proper lighting, tables, and linen. Gather all equipment you will need for a complete physical examination, and make sure you are familiar with its mechanical operation. You will not use all equipment today, but you will use it during the course of the semester, and this is the time to have it checked out.

Practice the steps of gathering data for a general survey, for height and weight, and vital signs on a peer. Record your findings using the regional write-up sheet that follows. The first section of the sheet is intended as a worksheet. It includes points for you to note that add up to the general survey. The bottom of the sheet has instructions for you to write the general survey statement; the topic sentence that will serve as an introduction for the complete physical examination writeup (see Jarvis, 2nd ed., p. 207 for an example).

NOTES

REGIONAL WRITE-UP—GENERAL SURVEY, VITAL SIGNS

Date _____

Client _____ Age _____ Sex ____ Occupation _____

Examiner _____

Physical Examination
General Survey
1. Physical appearance
   Age _____
   Gender _____
   Level of consciousness _____
   Skin color _____
   Facial features _____

2. Body structure
   Stature _____
   Nutrition _____
   Symmetry _____
   Posture _____
   Position _____
   Body build, contour _____
   Any physical deformity _____

3. Mobility
   Gait _____
   Range of motion _____

4. Behavior
   Facial expression _____
   Mood and affect _____
   Speech _____
   Dress _____
   Personal hygiene _____

Measurement
1. Height _____ cm _____ ft/in

2. Weight _____ kg _____ lb

Vital Signs
1. Temperature _____
2. Pulse
   Rate _____
   Rhythm _____
3. Respirations _____
4. Blood pressure _____ R arm _____ L arm

Summary
(Write a summary of the general survey, including height, weight, and vital signs. This will serve as an introduction for the complete physical examination writeup.)

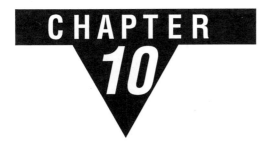

CHAPTER 10

Skin, Hair, and Nails

Purpose: This chapter helps you to learn the structure and function of the skin and its appendages; to understand the rationale for and the methods of inspection and palpation of the skin; and to record the assessment accurately.

Reading Assignment: Jarvis, *Physical Examination and Health Assessment*, 2nd ed., Chapter 10, pp. 214-265

_____

Audio-Visual Assignment: _____

_____

Glossary: Study the following terms after completing the reading assignment. You should be able to cover the definition on the right and define the term out loud.

Alopecia	(baldness) hair loss
Annular	circular shape to skin lesion
Bulla	elevated cavity containing free fluid larger than 1 cm diameter
Confluent	skin lesions that run together
Crust	thick dried out exudate left on skin when vesicles/pustules burst or dry up
Cyanosis	dusky blue color to skin or mucus membranes due to increased amount of unoxygenated hemoglobin
Erosion	scooped out, shallow depression in skin
Erythema	intense redness of the skin due to excess blood in dilated superficial capillaries, as in fever or inflammation
Excoriation	self-inflicted abrasion on skin due to scratching
Fissure	linear crack in skin extending into dermis
Furuncle	(boil) suppurative inflammatory skin lesion due to infected hair follicle
Hemangioma	skin lesion due to benign proliferation of blood vessels in the dermis
Iris	target shape of skin lesion

Jaundice   ....   yellow color to skin, palate, and sclera due to excess bilirubin in the blood

Keloid   ....   hypertrophic scar, elevated beyond site of original injury

Lichenification ....   tightly packed set of papules that thickens skin, from prolonged intense scratching

Lipoma   ....   benign fatty tumor

Maceration ....   softening of tissue by soaking

Macule   ....   flat skin lesion with only a color change

Nevus   ....   (mole) circumscribed skin lesion due to excess melanocytes

Nodule   ....   elevated skin lesion, > 1 cm diameter

Pallor   ....   excessively pale, whitish-pink color to lightly pigmented skin

Papule   ....   palpable skin lesion of < 1 cm diameter

Plaque   ....   skin lesion in which papules coalesce or come together

Pruritis   ....   itching

Purpura   ....   red-purple skin lesion due to blood in tissues from breaks in blood vessels

Pustule   ....   elevated cavity containing thick turbid fluid

Scale   ....   compact desiccated flakes of skin from shedding of dead skin cells

Telangiectasia ....   skin lesion due to permanently enlarged and dilated blood vessels that are visible

Ulcer   ....   sloughing of necrotic inflammatory tissue causes a deep depression in skin, extending into dermis

Vesicle   ....   elevated cavity containing free fluid up to 1 cm diameter

Wheal   ....   raised red skin lesion due to interstitial fluid

Zosteriform ....   linear shape of skin lesion along a nerve route

STUDY GUIDE

After completing the reading assignment and the audio-visual assignment, you should be able to answer the following questions in the spaces provided.

1. List the 3 layers associated with the skin, and describe the contents of each layer.

2. Define 2 types of human hair.

3. Differentiate between sebaceous, eccrine, and apocrine glands.

4. List at least 5 functions of the skin.

5. List at least 6 variables that are external to the skin itself that can influence skin color.

6. Describe the appearance of pallor, erythema, cyanosis, and jaundice, both in light-skinned and in dark-skinned persons. State common causes of each.

7. List causes of changes in skin temperature, texture, moisture, mobility, and turgor.

8. Describe each grade on the 4-point grading scale for pitting edema.

9. Distinguish the terms *primary* vs. *secondary* in reference to skin lesions.

10. The white linear markings that normally are visible through the nail and on the pink nail bed are termed_____.

11. Describe the following findings that are common variations on the infant's skin:

Mongolian spot_____

Café au lait spot _____

Erythema toxicum _____

Cutis marmorata _____

Physiologic jaundice _____

Milia _____

12. Describe the following findings that are common variations on the aging adult's skin:

Lentigines _____

Seborrheic keratosis _____

Actinic keratosis _____

Acrochordons (Skin tags)_____

Sebaceous hyperplasia _____

13. Differentiate between these purpuric lesions: petechiae; ecchymosis; hematoma.

14. Differentiate between the appearance of the skin rash of these childhood illnesses: measles (rubeola); German measles (rubella); chicken pox (varicella).

15. List and describe 3 skin lesions associated with AIDS.

16. Contrast a furuncle with an abscess.

17. Describe the appearance of these conditions of the nails: koilonychia; paronychia; Beau's line; splinter hemorrhages; onycholysis; clubbing.

18. Define and give an example of the following primary skin lesions: macule; papule; plaque; nodule; tumor; wheal; vesicle; pustule;

and of these secondary lesions: crust; scale; fissure; erosion; ulcer; excoriation; scar; atrophic scar; lichenification; keloid.

Fill in the labels indicated on the following illustrations.

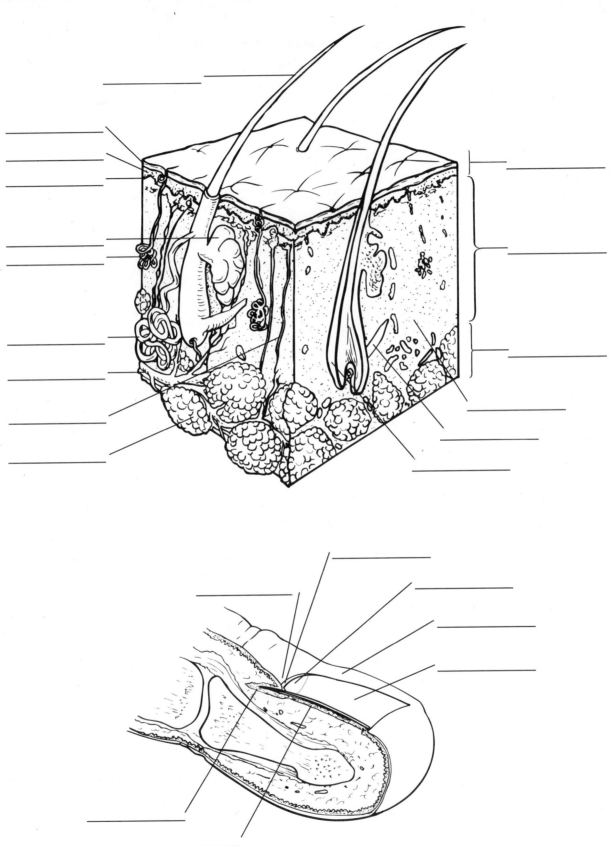

REVIEW QUESTIONS

This test is for you and is intended to check your own mastery of the content. Answers are provided in Appendix A.

1. Select the best description of the secretion of the eccrine glands.

   a) thick, milky
   b) dilute saline solution
   c) protective lipid substance
   d) keratin

2. Nevus is the medical term for

   a) a freckle.
   b) a birthmark.
   c) an infected hair follicle.
   d) a mole.

3. To assess for jaundice, the practitioner will assess the:

   a) sclera and mucous membranes.
   b) nails beds.
   c) lips.
   d) all visible skin surfaces.

4. Checking for skin temperature is best accomplished by using:

   a) palmar surface of the hands.
   b) ventral surface of the hands.
   c) fingertips.
   d) dorsal surface of the hands.

5. Skin turgor is assessed by picking up a large fold of skin on the anterior chest under the clavicle. This part of the examination is done to determine the presence of:

   a) edema.
   b) dehydration.
   c) Vitiligo.
   d) Scleroderma.

6. A lesion has been noted on a client during an examination. Select the description that is most complete.

   a) raised, irregular lesion, the size of a quarter, located on dorsum of left hand
   b) open lesion with no drainage or odor approximately 1/4 inch in diameter
   c) pedunculated lesion below left scapula with consistent red color. no drainage or odor
   d) dark brown, raised lesion, with irregular border, on dorsum of right foot, 3 cm in size with no drainage

7. Nail beds should be examined for clubbing. The normal angle between the nail base and the nails is:

   a) 100°
   b) 140°
   c) 160°
   d) 180°

8. The capillary beds should refill after being depressed in:

   a) < 1 second.
   b) > 2 second.
   c) 1–2 seconds.
   d) time is not significant as long as color returns.

9. During a routine visit, your client, aged 78, asks about small, flat, brown macules on the hands. Your best response after examining the areas is:

   a) "These are the result of sun exposure and do not require treatment."
   b) "These are related to exposure to the sun. We will examine them for any changes."
   c) "These are the skin tags that occur with aging. No treatment is required."
   d) "I'm glad you brought this to my attention. I will arrange for a biopsy."

Match column A to column B - items in column B may be used more than once

Column A—descriptor	Column B—skin layer
10. ___ basal cell layer	a) epidermis
11. ___ aids protection by cushioning	b) dermis
12. ___ collagen	c) subcutaneous layer
13. ___ adipose tissue	
14. ___ uniformly thin	
15. ___ stratum corneum	
16. ___ elastic tissue	

Column A—descriptor

Column B—color change

17. ___ pallor

18. ___ erythema

19. ___ cyanosis

20. ___ jaundice

a) intense redness of the skin due to excess blood in the dilated superficial capillaries

b) bluish mottled color that signifies decreased perfusion

c) absence of red-pink tones from the oxygenated hemoglobin in blood

d) increase in bilirubin in the blood causing a yellow color in the skin

Column A—descriptor

Column B—skin color change

21. ___ tiny, punctate red macules and papules on the cheeks, trunk, chest back and buttocks

22. ___ lower half of body turns red, upper half blanches

23. ___ transient mottling in trunk and extremities

24. ___ bluish color around the lips, hands and fingernails, and feet & toenails

25. ___ large round or oval patch of light brown pigmentation, usually present at birth.

26. ___ yellowing of skin, sclera, and mucous membranes due to increased numbers or red blood cells hemolyzed following birth

27. ___ yellow-orange color in light-skinned persons from large amounts of foods containing carotene

a)   Harlequin

b)   erythema toxicum

c)   acrocyanosis

d)   physiologic jaundice

e)   carotenemia

f)   café au lait

g)   cutis marmorata

SKILLS LABORATORY/CLINICAL SETTING

You are now ready for the clinical component of the integumentary system. Usually the clinical examination of the integumentary system is performed along with the examination of each particular body region. The purpose of practicing the steps of this examination separately is that you begin to think of the skin and its appendages as a separate organ system, and that you learn the components of skin examination.

Clinical Objectives

1. Inspect and palpate the skin, noting its color, vascularity, edema, moisture, temperature, texture, thickness, mobility and turgor, and any lesions.

2. Inspect the fingernails, noting color, shape, and any lesions.

3. Inspect the hair, noting texture, distribution, any lesions.

4. Record the history and physical examination findings accurately, reach an assessment of the health state, and develop a plan of care.

Instructions

Prepare the examination setting. Wash your hands. Practice the steps of the exam on a peer in the skills laboratory, giving appropriate instructions as you proceed. Choosing a peer from an ethnic background other than your own will further heighten your recognition of the range of normal skin tones. Record your findings using the regional write-up sheet that follows. The front of the page is intended as a worksheet; the back of the page is intended for your narrative summary recording using the SOAP format.

NOTES

REGIONAL WRITE-UP—SKIN, HAIR, AND NAILS

Date _____

Client_____ Age _____ Sex _____ Occupation _____

Examiner_____

I. Health History

	No	Yes, explain
1. Any previous **skin disease**?		
2. Any change in skin color or **pigmentation**?		
3. Any changes in a **mole**?		
4. Excessive **dryness** or **moisture**?		
5. Any skin **itching**?		
6. Any excess **bruising**?		
7. Any skin **rash** or **lesions**?		
8. Taking any **medications**?		
9. Any recent hair loss?		
10. Any change in nails?		
11. Any environmental hazards for skin?		
12. How do you take care of skin?		

II. Physical Examination

A. Inspect and palpate skin:

Color _____

Pigmentation _____

Temperature _____

Moisture _____

Texture _____

Thickness _____

Any edema _____

Mobility and turgor _____

Hygiene _____

Vascularity or Bruising _____

Any lesions _____

B. Inspect and palpate hair:

Color _____

Texture _____

Distribution _____

Any lesions _____

C. Inspect and palpate nails:

Shape and contour _____

Consistency _____

Color _____

D. Teach Skin Self-Examination

REGIONAL WRITE-UP—SKIN, HAIR, AND NAILS

Summarize your findings using the SOAP format.

Subjective (Client's reason for seeking care, health history)

Objective (Physical exam findings)   Record distribution of rash or lesions below

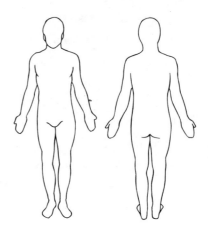

Assessment (Assessment of problem, diagnosis)

Plan (Diagnostic evaluation, follow-up care, teaching)

PERFORMANCE CHECKLIST

TEACHING SKIN SELF-EXAMINATION

	S	U	Comments
I. Cognitive			
1. Explain:			
a. Why skin is examined			
b. Who should perform skin self-examination			
c. Frequency of skin exam			
2. Define the ABCD rule			
3. Describe any equipment the client may need			
II. Performance			
1. Explains to client need for SSE			
2. Instructs client on technique of SSE by:			
a. demonstrating the order and body positioning for inspecting skin			
b. describing normal skin characteristics			
c. describing abnormal findings to look for			
3. Instructs client to report unusual findings to nurse or physician at once			

CHAPTER 11

Head and Neck, Including Regional Lymphatics

Purpose: This chapter helps you to learn the location and function of structures in the head and neck; to learn to perform inspection and palpation of the head and neck; and to record the assessment accurately.

Reading Assignment: Jarvis, *Physical Examination and Health Assessment*, 2nd ed., Chapter 11, pp. 268-297

_____

Audio-Visual Assignment: _____

_____

Glossary: Study the following terms after completing the reading assignment. You should be able to cover the definition on the right and define the term out loud.

Bruit	blowing swooshing sound heard through the stethoscope over an area of abnormal blood flow
Goiter	increase in size of thyroid gland that occurs with hyperthyroidism
Lymphadenopathy	enlargement of the lymph nodes due to infection, allergy, or neoplasm
Macrocephalic	abnormally large head
Microcephalic	abnormally small head
Normocephalic	round symmetric skull that is appropriately related to body size
Torticollis	head tilt due to congenital shortening or spasm of one sternomastoid muscle

STUDY GUIDE

After completing the reading assignment and the audio-visual assignment, you should be able to answer the following questions in the spaces provided.

1. The major neck muscles are the _____ and

   _____.

2. Name the borders of two regions in the neck, the anterior triangle, and the posterior triangle.

3. List the facial structures that should appear symmetric when inspecting the head.

4. Describe the characteristics of lymph nodes often associated with:

   acute infection

   chronic inflammation

   cancer

5. Differentiate *caput succedaneum* from *cephalhematoma* in the newborn infant.

6. Describe the tonic neck reflex in the infant.

7. Describe the characteristics of normal cervical lymph nodes during childhood.

8. List the condition(s) associated with parotid gland enlargement.

9. Describe the facial characteristics that occur with Down syndrome.

10. Contrast the facial characteristics of hyperthyroidism vs. hypothyroidism.

Fill in the labels indicated on the following illustrations.

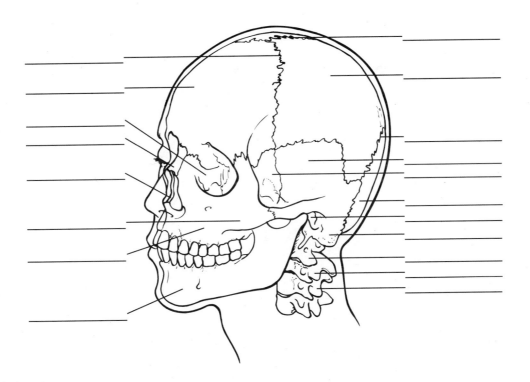

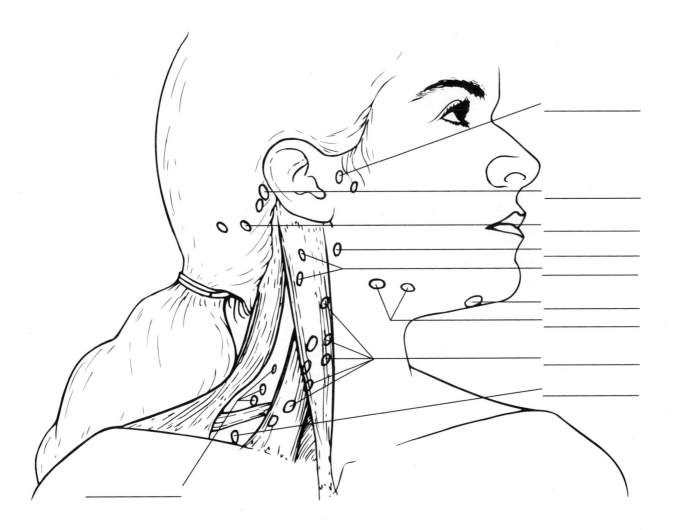

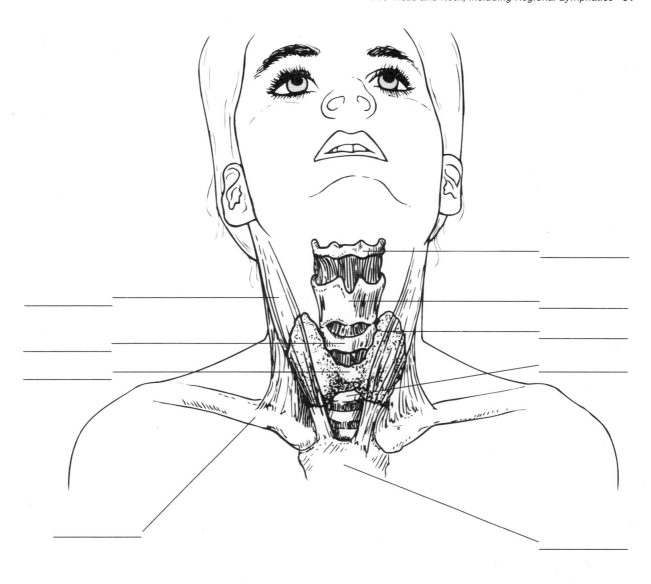

REVIEW QUESTIONS

This test is for you and is intended to check your own mastery of the content. Answers are provided in Appendix A.

1. Identify the facial bone that articulates at a joint instead of a suture.

    a.   zygomatic
    b.   maxilla
    c.   nasal
    d.   mandible.

2. Identify the blood vessel that runs diagonally across the sternomastoid muscle.

    a.   Temporal artery
    b.   Carotid artery
    c.   External jugular vein
    d.   Internal jugular vein

3. During the palpation of the lymphatics in the neck, palpable superficial cervical nodes are identified. The examiner should next examine:

   a.   the supraclavicular nodes.
   b.   the preauricular nodes.
   c.   the posterior cervical nodes.
   d.   the posterior auricular nodes.

4. Select the statement that is true regarding cluster headaches.

   a.   May be precipitated by alcohol and day-time napping
   b.   Usual occurrence is two per month each lasting 1 to 3 days
   c.   Characterized as throbbing
   d.   Tend to be supraorbital, retro-orbital or frontotemporal

5. Select the symptom that is least likely to indicate a possible malignancy.

   a.   History of radiation therapy to head, neck, or upper chest.
   b.   History of using chewing tobacco.
   c.   History of large alcohol consumption.
   d.   Tenderness.

6. Providing resistance while the client shrugs the shoulders is a test of the status of cranial nerve:

   a.   II
   b.   V
   c.   IX
   d.   XI

7. Upon examination, the fontanels should feel:

   a.   tense or bulging.
   b.   depressed or sunken.
   c.   firm, slightly concave and well defined.
   d.   pulsating.

Match column A to with column B

Column A—lymph nodes

8.   ___   Preauricular

9.   ___   Posterior auricular (mastoid)

10. ___   Occipital

11. ___   Submental

12. ___   Submaxillary (submandibular)

13. ___   Jugulodigastric

14. ___   Superficial cervical

15. ___   Deep cervical

16. ___   Posterior cervical

17. ___   Supraclavicular

Column B - location

a)   above and behind the clavicle

b)   deep under the sternomastoid muscle

c)   in front of the ear

d)   in the posterior triangle along the edge of the trapezius muscle

e)   superficial to the mastoid process

f)   at the base of the skull

g)   half way between the angle and the tip of the mandible

h)   behind the tip of the mandible

i)   under the angle of the mandible

j)   overlying the sternomastoid muscle

18. Cephalhematoma is associated with:

    a.   subperiosteal hemorrhage.

    b.   craniotabes.

    c.   bossing.

    d.   congenital syphilis.

SKILLS LABORATORY/ CLINICAL SETTING

You are now ready for the clinical component of the head and neck chapter. The purpose of the clinical component is to practice the steps of the head and neck examination on a peer in the skills laboratory and to achieve the following.

Clinical Objectives

1. Collect a health history related to pertinent signs and symptoms of the head and neck.

2. Inspect and palpate the skull noting size, contour, lumps, or tenderness.

3. Inspect the face noting facial expression, symmetry, skin characteristics, lesions.

4. Inspect and palpate the neck for symmetry, range of motion, and integrity of lymph nodes, trachea, and thyroid gland.

5. Record the findings systematically, reach an assessment of the health state, and develop a plan of care.

Instructions

Prepare the examination setting. Wash your hands. Practice the steps of the exam on a peer in the skills laboratory, giving appropriate instructions as you proceed. Record your findings using the regional write-up sheet that follows. The front of the page is intended as a worksheet; the back of the page is intended for your narrative summary recording using the SOAP format.

NOTES

REGIONAL WRITE-UP—HEAD AND NECK

Date _____

Client _____ Age _____ Sex ___ Occupation _____

Examiner _____

I. Health History

	No	Yes, explain
1. Any unusually frequent or unusually severe **headaches**?	_____	_____
2. Any **head injury**?	_____	_____
3. Experienced any **dizziness**?	_____	_____
4. Any neck **pain**?	_____	_____
5. Any **lumps** or **swelling** in head or neck?	_____	_____
6. Any surgery on head or neck?	_____	_____

II. Physical Examination

A. Inspect and palpate the skull

General size and contour _____

Deformities, lumps, tenderness _____

Temporal artery _____

Temporomandibular joint _____

B. Inspect the face

Facial expression _____

Symmetry of structures _____

Involuntary movements _____

Edema _____

Masses or lesions _____

Color and texture of skin _____

C. Inspect the neck

Symmetry _____

Range of motion, active _____

Test strength of cervical muscles _____

Abnormal pulsations _____

Enlargement of thyroid _____

Enlargement of lymph and salivary glands _____

D. Palpate the lymph nodes

Exact location _____

Size and shape _____

Presence or absence of tenderness _____

Freely movable, adherent to deeper structures, or matted together

Presence of surrounding inflammation _____

Texture (hard, soft, firm) _____

E. Palpate the trachea

F. Palpate the thyroid gland

G. Ausculate the thyroid gland (if enlarged)

REGIONAL WRITE-UP—HEAD AND NECK

Summarize your findings using the SOAP format.

Subjective (Client's reason for seeking care, health history)

Objective (Physical exam findings)

Assessment (Assessment of health state or problem, diagnosis)

Plan (Diagnostic evaluation, follow-up care, client teaching)

CHAPTER 12

Eyes

Purpose: This chapter helps you to learn the structure and function of the external and internal components of the eyes; to learn the methods of examination of vision, external eye, and ocular fundus; and to record the assessment accurately.

Reading Assignment: Jarvis, *Physical Examination and Health Assessment*, 2nd ed.,

Chapter 12, pp. 300-349

_____

Audio-Visual Assignment: _____

_____

Glossary: Study the following terms after completing the reading assignment. You should be able to cover the definition on the right and define the term out loud.

Accommodation .... adaptation of the eye for near vision by increasing the curvature of the lens

Anisocoria .... unequal pupil size

Arcus senilis .... gray-white arc or circle around the limbus of the iris that is common with aging

Argyll Robertson pupil .... pupil does not react to light; does constrict with accommodation

Astigmatism............................ refractive error of vision due to differences in curvature in refractive surfaces of the eye (cornea and lens)

A-V crossing............................ crossing paths of an artery and vein in the ocular fundus

Bitemporal hemianopsia........... loss of both temporal visual fields

Blepharitis .... inflammation of the glands and eyelash follicles along the margin of the eyelids

Cataract   .... opacity of the lens of the eye that develops slowly with aging and gradually obstructs vision

Chalazion .... infection or retention cyst of a meibomian gland, showing as a beady nodule on the eyelid

Conjunctivitis .... infection of the conjunctiva, "pink eye"

Cotton-wool area .... abnormal soft exudates visible as gray-white areas on the ocular fundus

Cup-disc ratio .... ratio of the width of the physiologic cup to the width of the optic disc, normally 1/2 or less

Diopter .... unit of strength of the lens settings on the ophthalmoscope that changes focus on the eye structures

Diplopia .... double vision

Drusen .... benign deposits on the ocular fundus that show as round yellow dots and occur commonly with aging

Ectropion .... lower eyelid loose and rolling outward

Entropion .... lower eyelid rolling inward

Exopthalmos .... protruding eyeballs

Fovea .... area of keenest vision at the center of the macula on the ocular fundus

Glaucoma .... a group of eye diseases characterized by increased intraocular pressure

Hordeolum .... (sty) red, painful pustule that is a localized infection of hair follicle at eyelid margin

Lid lag .... the abnormal white rim of sclera visible between the upper eyelid and the iris when a person moves the eyes downward

Macula .... round darker area of the ocular fundus that mediates vision only from the central visual field

Microaneurysm .... abnormal finding of round red dots on the ocular fundus that are localized dilatations of small vessels

Miosis .... constricted pupils

Mydriasis .... dilated pupils

Myopia .... "nearsighted," refractive error in which near vision is better than far vision

Nystagmus .... involuntary, rapid, rhythmic movement of the eyeball

Optic atrophy .... pallor of the optic disc due to partial or complete death of optic nerve

Optic disc .... area of ocular fundus in which blood vessels exit and enter

OD .... oculus dexter or right eye

OS .... oculus sinister or left eye

Papilledema .... stasis of blood flow out of the ocular fundus; sign of increased intracranial pressure

Presbyopia .... decrease in power of accomodation that occurs with aging

Pterygium .... triangular opaque tissue on the nasal side of the conjunctiva that grows toward the center of the cornea

Ptosis .... drooping of upper eyelid over the iris and possibly covering pupil

Red reflex .... red glow that appears to fill the person's pupil when first visualized through the ophthalmoscope

Strabismus .... (squint, crossed eye) disparity of the eye axes

Xanthelasma .... soft, raised yellow plaques occurring on the skin at the inner corners of the eyes

STUDY GUIDE

After completing the reading assignment and the audio-visual assignment, you should be able to answer the following questions in the spaces provided.

1. Name the 6 sets of extraocular muscles and the cranial nerve that innervates each one.

2. Name the 3 concentric coats of the eyeball.

3. Name the functions of the ciliary body, the pupil, and the iris.

4. Describe the compartments of the eye.

5. Describe how an image formed on the retina compares with its actual appearance in the outside world.

6. Describe the lacrimal system.

7. Define pupillary light reflex, fixation, and accomodation.

8. Concerning the pupillary light reflex, describe and contrast a direct light reflex with a consensual light reflex.

9. Identify common age-related changes in the eye.

10. Discuss the most common causes of decreased visual function in the older adult.

11. Explain the statement that normal visual acuity is 20/20.

12. Describe the method of testing for presbyopia.

13. To test for accomodation, the person focuses on a distant object, then shifts the gaze to a near object about 6 inches away. As near distance, you would expect the pupils to_____ (dilate/constrict), and the axes of the eyes to_____.

14. Concerning malalignment of the eye axes, contrast phoria with tropia.

15. Describe abnormal findings of tissue color that are possible on the conjunctiva and sclera, and their significance.

16. Describe the method of everting the upper eyelid for examination.

17. Contrast *pinguecula* with *pterygium*.

18. Contrast the use of the negative diopter or red lens settings with the positive diopter or black lens settings on the ophthalmoscope.

19. Contrast a *scleral crescent* with a *pigment crescent*.

20. Explain the rationale for testing for strabismus during early childhood.

21. Describe these findings and explain their significance: epicanthal fold; pseudostrabismus; Mongolian slant; opthalmia neonatorum; Brushfield's spots.

22. Describe the following 4 types of "red eye" and explain their significance: conjunctivitis; subconjunctival hemorrhage; iritis; acute glaucoma.

Fill in the labels indicated on the following illustrations.

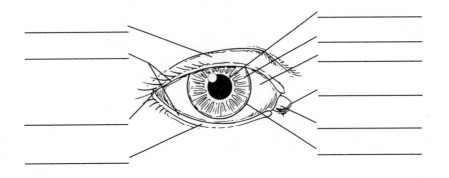

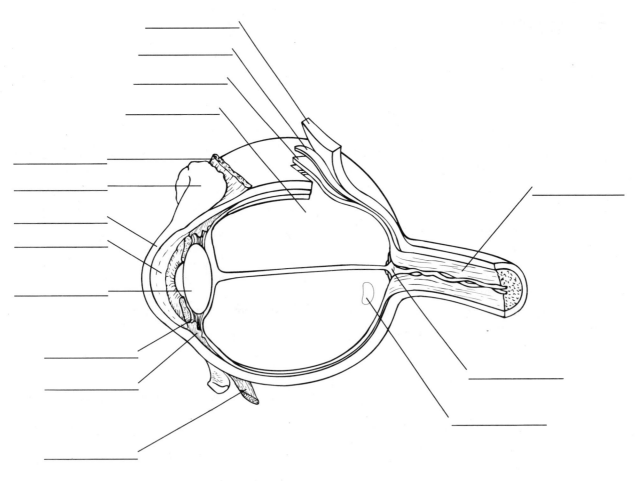

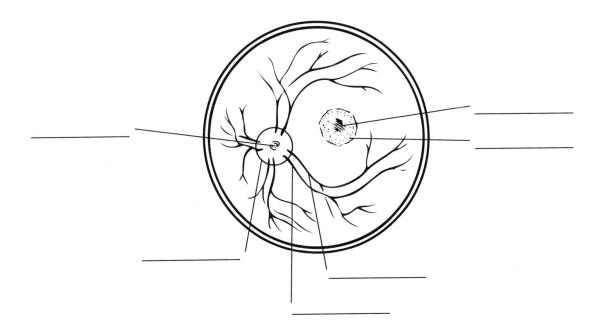

REVIEW QUESTIONS

This test is for you and is intended to check your own mastery of the content. Answers are provided in Appendix A.

1. The palpebral fissure is:

   a) the border between the cornea and sclera.
   b) the open space between the eyelids.
   c) the angle where the eyelids meet.
   d) visible on the upper and lower lids at the inner canthus.

2. The corneal reflex is mediated by cranial nerves:

   a) II & III.
   b) II & VI.
   c) V & VII.
   d) VI & IV.

3. The retinal structures viewed through the ophthalmoscope are:

   a) the optic disc, the retinal vessels, the general background, and the macula.
   b) the cornea, the lens, the choroid, and the ciliary body.
   c) the optic papilla, the sclera, the retina, and the iris.
   d) the pupil, the sclera, the ciliary body, and the macula.

4. The examiner records "positive consensual light reflex." This is:

   a) the convergence of the axes of the eyeballs.
   b) the simultaneous constriction of the other pupil when one eye is exposed to bright light.
   c) a reflex direction of the eye toward an object attracting a person's attention.
   d) the adaptation of the eye for near vision.

5. Several changes occur in the eye with the aging process. The thickening and yellowing of the lens is referred to as:

   a) presbyopia.
   b) floaters.
   c) macular degeneration.
   d) senile cataract.

6. The examiner must be alert to symptoms that may constitute an eye emergency. Identify the symptom(s) that should be referred immediately.

   a) diplopia, scotoma
   b) halos, epiphora
   c) sudden onset of vision change
   d) photophobia

7. Visual acuity is assessed with:

   a) the Snellen eye chart.
   b) an ophthalmoscope.
   c) the Hirschberg test.
   d) the confrontation test.

8. The cover test is used to assess for:

   a) nystagmus.
   b) peripheral vision.
   c) muscle weakness.
   d) extraocular muscle function.

9. The examiner is ready to use the ophthalmoscope. The examiner would:

   a) remove his or her own glasses and approach the client's left eye with his or her left eye.
   b) leave light on in the examining room and remove glasses from the client.
   c) remove glasses and set the diopter setting at 0.
   d) use the smaller white light and instruct the client to focus on the ophthalmoscope.

10. Briefly describe the method of assessing the six cardinal fields of vision.

SKILLS LABORATORY/ CLINICAL SETTING

You are now ready for the clinical component of the eye examination. The purpose of the clinical component is to practice the steps of the examination on a peer in the skills laboratory. Note that the first practice session usually takes a long time because there are so many separate steps. Be aware that success with the use of the ophthalmoscope is hard to achieve during the first practice session. Make sure you are holding the instrument correctly and practice focusing on various objects about the room before you try to look at a person's fundus. When you do examine a peer's eye, make sure to offer occasional rest times. It is very tiring for the "client" to have the ophthalmoscope light shining in the eye. During the first practice session, aim for finding the red reflex and a retinal vessel or two; if you can locate the optic disc, so much the better.

Clinical Objectives

1. Collect a health history related to pertinent signs and symptoms of the eye system.

2. Demonstrate and explain assessment of visual acuity, visual fields, external eye structures, ocular fundus.

3. Record the history and physical examination findings accurately, reach an assessment of the health state, and develop a plan of care.

Instructions

Prepare the examination setting. Wash your hands. Practice the steps of the exam on a peer in the skills laboratory, giving appropriate instructions as you proceed. Record your findings using the regional write-up sheet that follows. The front of the page is intended as a worksheet; the back of the page is intended for your narrative summary recording using the SOAP format.

NOTES

REGIONAL WRITE-UP—EYES

Date _____

Client_____ Age_____ Sex___ Occupation_____

Examiner_____

I. Health History

		No	Yes, explain
1.	Any **difficulty seeing** or blurring?	_____	_____
2.	Any eye **pain**?	_____	_____
3.	Any history of **crossed eyes**?	_____	_____
4.	Any **redness** or **swelling** in eyes?	_____	_____
5.	Any **watering** or **tearing**?	_____	_____
6.	Any **injury** or **surgery** to eye?	_____	_____
7.	Ever tested for **glaucoma**?	_____	_____
8.	Wear **glasses** or **contact lenses**?	_____	_____
9.	Ever had vision tested?	_____	_____
10.	Taking any medications?	_____	_____

II. Physical Examination

A. Test visual acuity
Snellen Eye chart _____
Pocket vision screener for near vision _____

B. Test Visual fields
Confrontation test _____

C. Inspect extraocular muscle function
Corneal light reflex _____
Cover test _____
Diagnostic positions test _____

D. Inspect external eye structures
General _____
Eyebrows_____
Eyelids and lashes _____
Eyeballs_____
Conjunctiva and sclera _____
Lacrimal gland, puncta _____

E. Inspect anterior eyeball structures
Cornea _____
Iris _____
Pupil size _____
Pupil direct and consensual light reflex _____
Accomodation _____

F. Inspect ocular fundus
Optic disc _____
Vessels _____
General background of fundus _____
Macula _____

REGIONAL WRITE-UP—EYES

Summarize your findings using the SOAP format.

Subjective (Client's reason for seeking care, health history)

Objective (Physical exam findings)   Record findings on diagram below

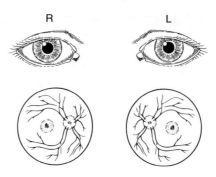

R   L

Assessment (Assessment of problem, diagnosis)

Plan (Diagnostic evaluation, follow-up care, teaching)

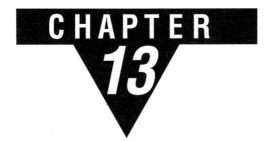

Ears

Purpose: This chapter helps you to learn the structure and function of the ears; to learn the methods of examination of hearing, external ear structures, and tympanic membrane using the otoscope; and to record the assessment accurately.

Reading Assignment: Jarvis, *Physical Examination and Health Assessment*, 2nd ed.,

Chapter 13, pp. 352-384

_____

Audio-Visual Assignment: _____

_____

Glossary: Study the following terms after completing the reading assignment. You should be able to cover the definition on the right and define the term out loud.

Annulus	outer fibrous rim encircling the eardrum
Atresia	congenital absence or closure of ear canal
Cerumen	yellow waxy material that lubricates and protects the ear canal
Cochlea	inner ear structure containing the central hearing apparatus
Eustachian Tube	connects the middle ear with the nasopharynx and allows passage of air
Helix	superior, posterior free rim of the pinna
Incus	"anvil," middle of the 3 ossicles of the middle ear
Malleus	"hammer," first of the 3 ossicles of the middle ear
Mastoid	bony prominence of the skull located just behind the ear
Organ of Corti	sensory organ of hearing
Otalgia	pain in the ear
Otitis externa	inflammation of the outer ear and ear canal
Otitis media	inflammation of the middle ear and tympanic membrane
Otorrhea	discharge from the ear

Pars flaccida .... small, slack, superior section of tympanic membrane

Pars tensa .... thick, taut, central/inferior section of tympanic membrane

Pinna   .... auricle, or outer ear

Stapes   .... "stirrup," inner of the 3 ossicles of the middle ear

Tinnitus   .... ringing in the ears

Tympanic membrane .... "eardrum," thin, translucent, oval membrane that stretches across the ear canal and separates the middle ear from the outer ear

Umbo   .... knob of the malleus that shows through the tympanic membrane

Vertigo   .... a spinning, twirling sensation

STUDY GUIDE

After completing the reading assignment and the audio-visual assignment, you should be able to answer the following questions in the spaces provided.

1. List the 3 functions of the middle ear.

2. Contrast 2 pathways of hearing.

3. Differentiate among the types of hearing loss, and give examples.

4. Relate the anatomic differences that place the infant at greater risk for middle ear infections.

5. Describe these tests of hearing acuity: voice test; Weber test; Rinne test.

6. Explain the positioning of normal ear alignment in the child.

7. Define *otosclerosis* and *presbycusis*.

8. Contrast the motions used to straighten the ear canal when using the otoscope with an infant vs. an adult.

9. Describe the appearance of these nodules that could be present on the external ear: Darwin's tubercle; sebaceous cyst; tophi; chondrodermatitis; keloid; carcinoma.

10. Describe the appearance of these conditions that could appear in the ear canal: osteoma; exostosis; furuncle; polyp; foreign body.

11. List the indications of the following descriptions of the appearance of the eardrum: yellow-amber color_____; pearly gray color_____; air fluid level_____; distorted light reflex_____; red color_____; dense white areas_____; oval dark areas_____; black or white dots on drum_____; blue drum _____.

12. List the findings that commonly appear during the Weber test and the Rinne test for:

conductive hearing loss _____

_____

sensorineural loss _____

_____

13. Fill in the labels indicated on the following illustrations.

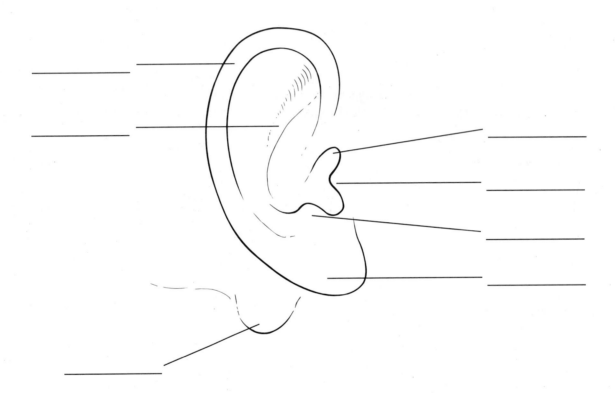

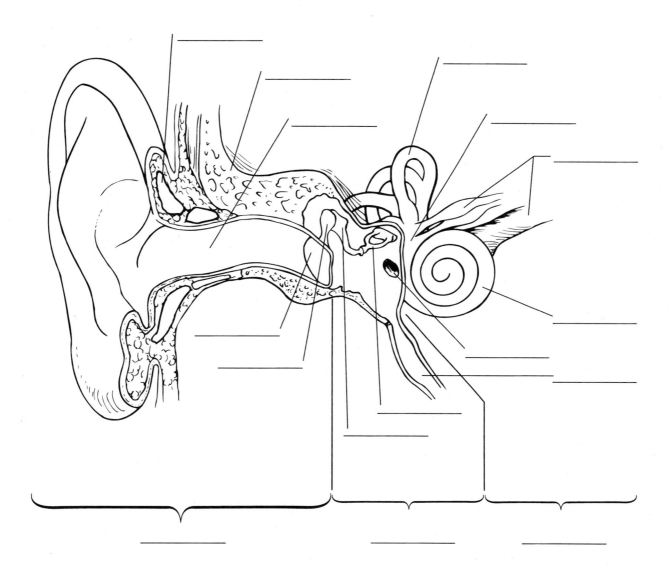

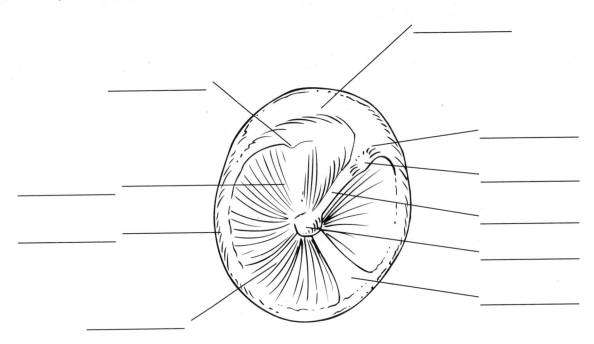

REVIEW QUESTIONS

This test is for you and is intended to check your own mastery of the content. Answers are provided in Appendix A.

1. Using the otoscope, the tympanic membrane is visualized. The color of a normal membrane is:

   a) deep pink.
   b) creamy white.
   c) pearly gray.
   d) dependent upon the ethnicity of the individual.

2. Sensorineural hearing loss is caused by:

   a) a gradual nerve degeneration.
   b) foreign bodies.
   c) impacted cerumen
   d) perforated tympanic membrane.

3. Prior to examining the ear with the otoscope, the ___ should be palpated for tenderness.

   a) Helix, external auditory meatus, and lobule
   b) Mastoid process, tympanic membrane and malleus
   c) Pinna, Pars flaccida and antitragus
   d) Pinna, tragus and mastoid process

4. During the otoscopic examination of a child less than 3 years of age, the examiner:

   a) pulls the pinna up and back.
   b) pulls the pinna down.
   c) holds the pinna gently but firmly in its normal position.
   d) tilts the head slightly toward the examiner.

5. While viewing with the otoscope, the examiner instructs the client to hold the nose and swallow. During this maneuver, the ear drum should:

   a) flutter.
   b) retract.
   c) bulge.
   d) remain immobile.

6. To differentiate between air conduction and bone conduction hearing loss, the examiner would perform:

   a) the Weber test.
   b) the Romberg test.
   c) the Rinne test.
   d) the whisper test.

7. During the examination of a child, the ear position is assessed. The ear should be positioned within _____ of the vertical.

   a) 5°
   b) 7°
   c) 10°
   d) 15°

8. During a chart review, the following notation is found: "Darwin's tubercle bilaterally." This is:

   a) an overgrowth of scar tissue.
   b) a blocked sebaceous gland.
   c) a sign of gout called tophi.
   d) a congenital, painless nodule at the helix.

SKILLS LABORATORY/ CLINICAL SETTING

You are now ready for the clinical component of the ear examination. The purpose of the clinical component is to practice the steps of the ear examination on a peer in the skills laboratory or on a client in the clinical setting. The use of the otoscope is somewhat easier than the use of the ophthalmoscope; however you still must be sure you are holding the instrument correctly. Holding the otoscope in an "upside down" position seems awkward at first, but it is important in order to make sure the otoscope tip does not cause pain to the delicate parts of the ear canal. Have someone correct your positioning before you insert the instrument.

Clinical Objectives

1. Collect a health history related to pertinent signs and symptoms of the ear system.

2. Describe the appearance of the normal outer ear and external ear canal.

3. Describe and demonstrate the correct technique of an otoscopic examination.

4. Describe and perform tests for hearing acuity.

5. Systematically describe the normal tympanic membrane including position, color, and landmarks.

6. Record the history and physical examination findings accurately, reach an assessment about the health state, and develop a plan of care.

Instructions

Prepare the examination setting and gather your equipment. Make certain the otoscope light is bright and batteries are freshly charged. Wash your hands. Practice the steps of the exam on a peer in the skills laboratory, giving appropriate instructions as you proceed. Record your findings using the regional write-up sheet that follows. The front of the page is intended as a worksheet; the back of the page is intended for your narrative summary recording using the SOAP format.

REGIONAL WRITE-UP—EARS

Date _____

Client _____ Age _____ Sex ____ Occupation _____

Examiner _____

I. Health History

		No	Yes, explain

1. Any **earache** or ear pain?
2. Any ear **infections**?
3. Any **discharge** from ears?
4. Any **hearing loss**?
5. Any **loud noises** at home or job?
6. Any **ringing** or buzzing in ears?
7. Ever felt **vertigo** (spinning)?
8. How do you clean your ears? _____

II. Physical Examination

A. Inspect and palpate external ear

Size and shape _____

Skin condition _____

Tenderness _____

External auditory meatus _____

B. Inspect using the otoscope

External canal _____

Tympanic membrane _____

   Color and characteristics _____

   Position _____

   Integrity of membrane _____

C. Test hearing Acuity

Voice test _____

Weber test _____

Rinne Test _____

REGIONAL WRITE-UP—EARS

Summarize your findings using the SOAP format.

Subjective (Client's reason for seeking care, health history)

Objective (Physical exam findings)   Record findings on diagram below

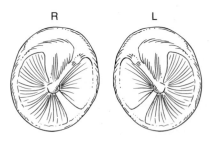

R   L

Assessment (Assessment of health state or problem, diagnosis)

Plan (Diagnostic evaluation, follow-up care, client teaching)

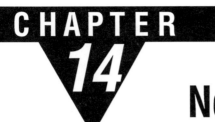

CHAPTER 14

Nose, Mouth, and Throat

Purpose: This chapter helps you to learn the structure and function of the nose, mouth, and throat; to learn the methods of inspection and palpation of these structures; and to record the assessment accurately.

Reading Assignment: Jarvis, *Physical Examination and Health Assessment*, 2nd ed.,

Chapter 14, pp. 386-423

Audio-Visual Assignment: _____

Glossary: Study the following terms after completing the reading assignment. You should be able to cover the definition on the right and define the term out loud.

Aphthous ulcers .... "canker sores"— small, painful, round ulcers in the oral mucosa of
unknown cause

Buccal   .... pertaining to the cheek

Candidiasis .... (Moniliasis) white, cheesy, curdlike patch on buccal mucosa due to
superficial fungal infection

Caries   .... decay in the teeth

Crypts   .... indentations on surface of tonsils

Cheilitis   .... red, scaling, shallow, painful fissures at corners of mouth

Choanal atresia .... closure of nasal cavity due to congenital septum between nasal
cavity and pharynx

Epistaxis   .... nosebleed, usually from anterior septum

Epulis   .... nontender, fibrous nodule of the gum

Fordyce's granules .... small, isolated, white or yellow papules on oral mucosa

Gingivitis .... red swollen gum margins that bleed eassily

Herpes simplex .... "cold sores"— clear vesicles with red base, evolve into pustules,
usually at lip-skin junction

Koplik's spots .... small blue-white spots with red halo over oral mucosa; early sign of measles

Leukoplakia .... chalky white, thick raised patch on sides of tongue; precancerous

Malocclusion .... upper or lower dental arches out of alignment

Papillae   .... rough bumpy elevation on dorsal surface of tongue

Parotid glands .... pair of salivary glands in the cheeks in front of the ears

Pharyngitis .... inflammation of the throat

Plaque   .... soft whitish debris on teeth

Polyp   .... smooth, pale gray nodules in the nasal cavity due to chronic allergic rhinitis

Rhinitis   .... red swollen inflammation of nasal mucosa

Thrush   .... oral candidiasis in the newborn

Turbinate   .... one of 3 bony projections into nasal cavity

Uvula   .... free projection hanging down from the middle of the soft palate

STUDY GUIDE

After completing the reading assignment and the audio-visual assignment, you should be able to answer the following questions in the spaces provided.

1. Name the functions of the nose.

2. Describe the size and components of the nasal cavity.

3. List the 4 sets of paranasal sinuses and describe their function.

4. List the 3 pairs of salivary glands, including their location and the locations of their duct openings.

5. Following tooth loss in the middle or older adult, describe the consequences of chewing with the remaining maloccluded teeth.

6. Describe the appearance of a deviated nasal septum, and a perforated septum.

7. Describe the appearance of a torus palatinus and explain its significance.

8. Contrast the physical appearance and clinical significance of: leukoedema; candidiasis; leukoplakia; Fordyce's granules.

9. List the 4 point grading scale for the size of tonsils.

10. Describe the appearance and clinical significance of these findings in the infant: sucking tubercle; Epstein's pearls; Bednar aphthae.

11. Constrast the appearance of nasal turbinates vs. nasal polyps.

12. Describe the appearance and clinical significance of these findings on the tongue: ankyloglossia; fissured tongue; geographic tongue; black hairy tongue; macroglossia.

13. In the space below, sketch a cleft palate and a bifid uvula.

14. Describe the appearance of oral Kaposi's sarcoma.

15. Fill in the labels indicated on the following illustrations.

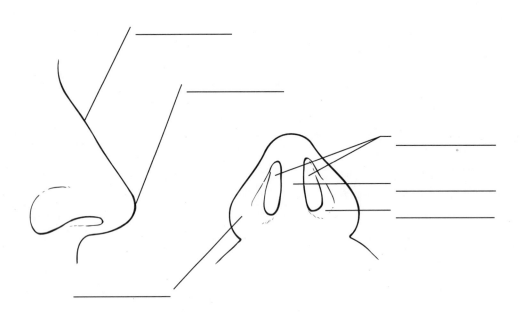

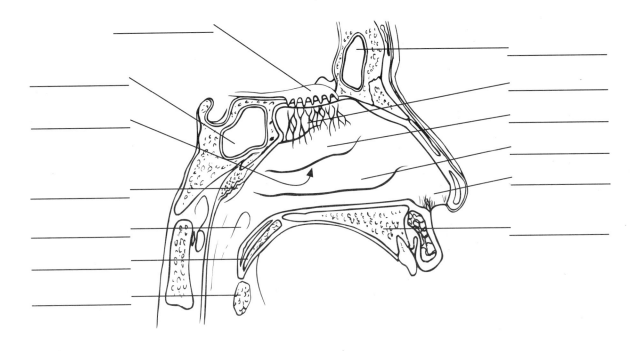

LEFT LATERAL WALL-NASAL CAVITY

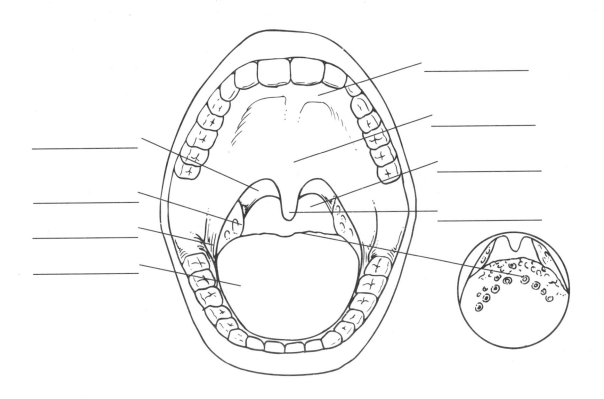

REVIEW QUESTIONS

This test is for you and is intended to check your own mastery of the content. Answers are provided in Appendix A.

1. The most common site of nosebleeds is:

   a.   the turbinates.
   b.   the collumella
   c.   Kiesselbach's plexus.
   d.   the meatus.

2. The sinuses that are accessible to examination are the:

   a.   ethmoid and sphenoid.
   b.   frontal and ethmoid.
   c.   maxillary and sphenoid.
   d.   frontal and maxillary sinuses.

3. The frenulum is:

   a.   the midline fold of tissue that connects the tongue to the floor of the mouth
   b.   the anterior border of the oral cavity.
   c.   the arching roof of the mouth.
   d.   the free projection hanging down from the middle of the soft palate.

4. The largest salivary gland is located:

   a.   within the cheeks in front of the ear.
   b.   beneath the mandible at the angle of the jaw.
   c.   within the floor of the mouth under the tongue.
   d.   at the base of the tongue.

5. A 70-year-old client complains of dry mouth. The most frequent cause of this problem is:

   a.   the aging process.
   b.   related to medications the client may be taking.
   c.   the use of dentures.
   d.   related to a diminished sense of smell.

6. Because the client has complained of headache, the examiner uses transillumination to assess for an inflamed sinus. The findings in a healthy individual would be:

   a.   a diffuse red glow.
   b.   no transillumination.
   c.   findings vary with ethnicity of the client.
   d.   light is visible in the nares through a speculum.

7. During an inspection of the nares, a deviated septum is noted. The best action is:

   a.   request a consultation with an ear, nose and throat specialist.
   b.   document the deviation in the medical record in case the client needs to be suctioned.
   c.   teach the client what to do if a nose bleed should occur.
   d.   explore further because polyps frequently accompany a deviated septum.

8. Oral malignancies are most likely to develop:

   a.   on the soft palate
   b.   on the tongue.
   c.   in the buccal cavity.
   d.   under the tongue.

9. In a medical record, the tonsils are graded as 3+. When the mouth of this client is examined, the tonsils would be:

   a.   visible.
   b.   halfway between tonsillar pillars and uvula.
   c.   touching the uvula.
   d.   touching each other.

SKILLS LABORATORY/CLINICAL SETTING

You are now ready for the clinical component of the nose, mouth, and throat examination. The purpose of the clinical component is to practice the steps of the examination on a peer in the skills laboratory or on a client in the clinical setting and to achieve the following.

Clinical Objectives

1. Inspect the external nose.

2. Demonstrate use of the otoscope and nasal attachment to inspect the structures of the nasal cavity.

3. Demonstrate knowledge of infection control practices during inspection and palpation of structures of the mouth and pharynx.

4. Record the history and physical examination findings accurately, reach an assessment of the health state, and develop a plan of care.

Instructions

Prepare the examination setting and gather your equipment. Wash your hands. Practice the steps of the exam on a peer in the skills laboratory, giving appropriate instructions as you proceed. Record your findings using the regional write-up sheet that follows. The front of the page is intended as a worksheet; the back of the page is intended for your narrative summary recording using the SOAP format.

NOTES

REGIONAL WRITE-UP—NOSE, MOUTH, AND THROAT

Date _____

Client _____ Age ____ Sex ___ Occupation _____

Examiner _____

I. Health History—Nose

		No	Yes, explain
1.	Any nasal **discharge**?	_____	_____
2.	Unusually frequent or severe colds?	_____	_____
3.	Any **sinus pain** or sinusitis?	_____	_____
4.	Any **trauma** or injury to nose?	_____	_____
5.	Any **nosebleeds**? How often?	_____	_____
6.	Any **allergies** or hay fever?	_____	_____
7.	Any change in sense of smell?	_____	_____

Mouth and Throat

1.	Any **sores** in mouth, tongue?	_____	_____
2.	Any **sore throat**? How often?	_____	_____
3.	Any **bleeding gums**?	_____	_____
4.	Any **toothache**?	_____	_____
5.	Any **hoarseness**, voice change?	_____	_____
6.	Any difficulty **swallowing**?	_____	_____
7.	Any change in sense of taste?	_____	_____
8.	Do you smoke? How much/day?	_____	_____
9.	Tell me about usual dental care.	_____	_____

II. Physical Examination

A. Inspect and palpate the nose

Symmetry _____

Deformity, asymmetry, inflammation _____

Test patency of each nostril _____

Using nasal speculum, note:

Color of nasal mucosa _____

Discharge, foreign body _____

Septum: deviation, perforation, bleeding _____

Turbinates: color, swelling, exudate, polyps _____

B. Palpate the sinus area

Frontal _____

Maxillary _____

Transillumination (if indicated) _____

C. Inspect the mouth

Lips _____

Teeth and gums _____

Buccal mucosa _____

Palate and uvula _____

D. Inspect the throat

Tonsils: condition and grade _____

Pharyngeal wall _____

Any breath odor _____

REGIONAL WRITE-UP—NOSE, MOUTH, AND THROAT

Summarize your findings using the SOAP format.

Subjective (Client's reason for seeking care, health history)

Objective (Physical exam findings)   Record findings on diagram below

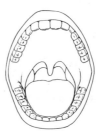

Assessment (Assessment of health state or problem, diagnosis)

Plan (Diagnostic evaluation, follow-up care, client teaching)

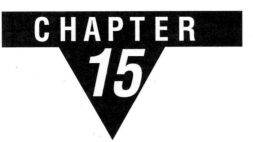

CHAPTER 15

Breasts and Regional Lymphatics

Purpose: This chapter helps you to learn the structure and function of the breast, to understand the rationale and methods of examination of the breast, to accurately record the assessment, and to teach breast self examination.

Reading Assignment: Jarvis, *Physical Examination and Health Assessment*, 2nd ed., Chapter 15, pp. 426-457

Audio-Visual Assignment: _____

Glossary: Study the following terms after completing the reading assignment. You should be able to cover the definition on the right and define the term out loud.

Alveoli .... smallest structure of mammary gland

Areola .... darkened area surrounding nipple

Colostrum .... thin, yellow fluid, precursor of milk, secreted a few days after birth

Cooper's ligaments .... suspensory ligament, fibrous bands extending from the inner breast surface to the chest wall muscles

Fibroadenoma .... benign breast mass

Gynecomastia .... excessive breast development in the male

Inverted .... nipples that are depressed or invaginated

Intraductal papilloma .... serosanguinous nipple discharge

Lactiferous .... conveying milk

Mastitis .... inflammation of the breast

Montgomery's glands .... sebaceous glands in the areola, secrete protective lipid during lactation. Also called Tubercles of Montgomery

Paget's disease .... intraductal carcinoma in the breast

Peau d'orange .... orange peel appearance of breast due to edema

Retraction .... dimple or pucker on the skin

Striae .... atrophic pink, purple or white linear streaks on the breasts, associated with pregnancy, excessive weight gain, or rapid growth during adolescence

Supernumerary nipple .... minute extra nipple along the embryonic milk line

Tail of Spence .... extension of breast tissue into the axilla

STUDY GUIDE

After completing the reading assignment and the audio-visual assignment, you should be able to answer the following questions in the spaces provided.

1. Identify appropriate history questions to ask a client regarding the breast exam.

2. Describe the anatomy of the breast.

3. Correlate changes in the female breast with normal developmental stages.

4. Describe the components of the breast exam.

5. List points to include in teaching the breast self exam.

6. Explain the significance of a supernumerary nipple/breast.

7. Differentiate between the female and male examination procedure and findings.

8. Discuss pathologic changes that may occur in the breast:

   benign breast disease

   abscess

   acute mastitis

   fibroadenoma

   cancer

   Paget's disease.

9. List and describe the characteristics to consider when a mass is noted in the breast.

10. Define gynecomastia.

11. Recall additional diagnostic techniques used for diagnosis of breast lesions.

12. List the high risk and moderate risk factors that increase the usual risk of breast cancer.

13. Fill in the labels on the following diagrams.

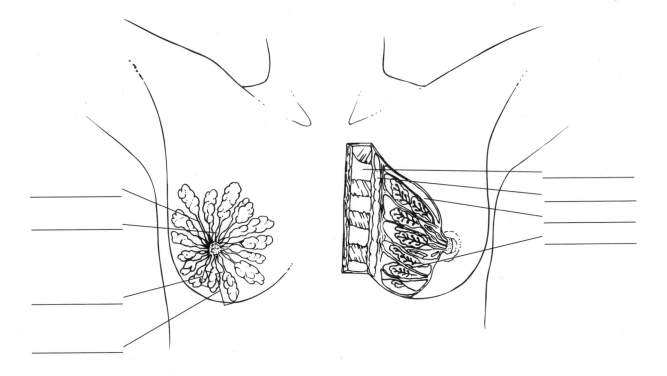

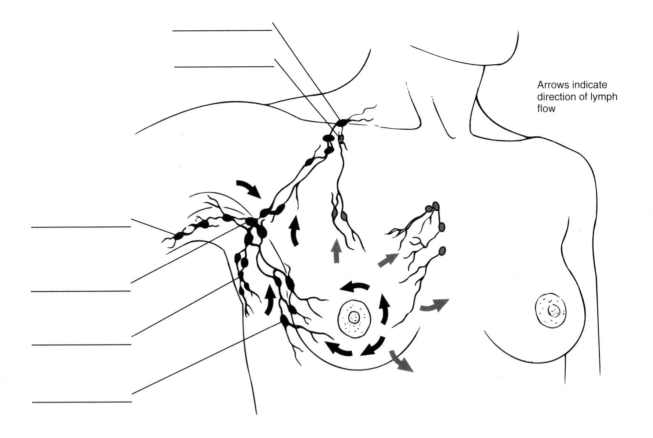

Arrows indicate
direction of lymph
flow

REVIEW QUESTIONS

This test is for you and is intended to check your own mastery of the content. Answers are provided
in Appendix A.

1. The reservoirs for storing milk in the breast are:

   a. lobules.
   b. alveoli.
   c. Montgomery's glands.
   d. lactiferous sinuses.

2. The most common site of breast tumors is:

   a. upper inner quadrant.
   b. upper outer quadrant.
   c. lower inner quadrant
   d. lower outer quadrant.

3. During a visit for a school physical, the 13-year-old girl being examined questions the asymmetry of her breasts. The best response is:

   a. "One breast may grow faster than the other during development."
   b. "I will give you a referral for a mammogram."
   c. "You will probably have fibrocystic disease when you are older."
   d. "This may be an indication of hormonal imbalance. We will check again in 6 months."

4. When instructing a client about self breast exam, you would inform the client that the best time to conduct breast self-examination is:

    a. At the onset of the menstrual period.
    b. On the 14th day of the menstrual cycle.
    c. On the 4th to 7th day of the cycle.
    d. Just before the menstrual period.

5. This is the first visit for a female client, age 38. The practitioner instructs her that a baseline mammogram is recommended for women between the ages of 35 and 39 and that the exam schedule would be based on age. The recommendation for women 40 to 49 is:

    a. every year.
    b. every 1 to 2 years.
    c. twice a year.
    d. only the base line exam is needed unless the client has symptoms.

6. The examiner is going to inspect the breasts for retraction. The best position for this part of the exam is:

    a. lying supine with arms at the sides.
    b. leaning forward with hands outstretched.
    c. sitting with hand pushing onto hips.
    d. one arm at the side, the other arm elevated.

7. A bimanual technique may be the preferred approach for a client:

    a. who is pregnant.
    b. who is having the first breast exam by a health care provider
    c. with pendulous breasts.
    d. who has felt a change in the breast during self examination.

8. During the examination of a 70-year-old male client, gynecomastia is noted. The next action of the examiner would be to:

    a. refer the client for a biopsy.
    b. refer the client for a mammogram.
    c. review the client's medications for drugs that have gynecomastia as a side effect.
    d. proceed with the exam. This is normal part of the aging process.

9. During a breast examination, a mass is felt. Identify the description that is most consistent with cancer rather than benign breast disease.

    a. Round, firm, well demarcated.
    b. Irregular, poorly defined, fixed.
    c. Rubbery, mobile, tender.
    d. Lobular, clear margins, negative skin retraction.

10. During the examination of the breasts of a pregnant client, you would expect to find:

    a. Peau d'Orange.
    b. nipple retraction.
    c. a unilateral, obvious venous pattern.
    d. a blue vascular pattern over both breasts.

SKILLS LABORATORY/ CLINICAL SETTING

You are now ready for the clinical component of the breast assessment. The purpose of the clinical component is to practice the steps of the assessment on a peer in the skills laboratory and to achieve the following.

Clinical Objectives

1. Demonstrate knowledge of the symptoms related to the breasts and axillae by obtaining a health history from a client.

2. Perform inspection and palpation of the breasts, with the client in sitting and supine positions, using proper technique and providing appropriate draping.

3. Teach the breast self exam to a client or list the points to include in teaching the breast self exam.

4. Record the history and physical exam findings accurately, reach an assessment of the health state, and develop a plan of care.

Instructions

Practice the steps of the breast exam on a peer or on a client in the clinical area. Record your findings on the regional write-up sheet that follows.

NOTES

REGIONAL WRITE-UP—BREASTS AND AXILLAE

Date _____

Client_____ Age _____ Sex ___ Occupation _____

Examiner_____

I. Health History

	No	Yes, explain
1. Any **pain** or tenderness in breasts?		
2. Any **lump** or thickening in breasts?		
3. Any **discharge** from nipples?		
4. Any **rash** on breasts?		
5. Any **swelling** in the breasts?		
6. Any **trauma** or injury to breasts?		
7. Any **history** of breast disease?		
8. Ever had **surgery** on breasts?		
9. Ever been taught breast self-exam?		
10. Ever had mammography?		

II. Physical Examination

A. Inspection

1. Breasts
   Symmetry _____
   Skin color and condition _____
   Texture _____
   Lesions _____

2. Areolae and nipples
   Shape _____
   Direction _____
   Surface characteristics _____
   Discharge _____

3. Response to arm movement _____

4. Axillae _____

B. Palpation

1. Breasts
   Texture _____
   Masses _____
   Tenderness _____

2. Areolae and nipples
   Masses _____
   Discharge _____

3. Axillae and lymph nodes
   Size _____
   Shape _____
   Consistency _____
   Mobility _____
   Discrete or matted _____
   Tenderness _____

C. Teach breast self exam

REGIONAL WRITE-UP—BREASTS AND AXILLAE

Summarize your findings using the SOAP format.

Subjective (Client's reason for seeking care, health history)

Objective (Physical exam findings)   Record findings on diagram below

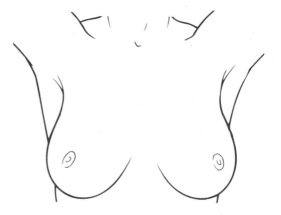

Assessment (Assessment of problem, diagnosis)

Plan (Diagnostic evaluation, follow-up care, teaching)

PERFORMANCE CHECKLIST

TEACHING BREAST EXAMINATION

	S	U	Comments
I. Cognitive			
1. Explain:			
a. Why breasts are examined			
(1) in the shower			
(2) before a mirror			
(3) supine with pillow under side of breast being examined			
b. who should do breast exam			
c. frequency of breast exam			
d. best time of month to do breast exam and rationale			
2. State the area of breast where most lumps are found			
3. Give two reasons a person may not report significant findings to their health care provider			
II. Performance			
1. Explains to client need for SBE			
2. Instructs client on technique of SBE by:			
a. inspecting and bilaterally comparing breasts in front of mirror			
b. palpating breast in a systemic manner, using pads of three fingers and with client's arm raised overhead			
c. palpating tail of spence and axilla			
d. gently compressing nipples			
3. Instructs client to report unusual findings to the physician at once			

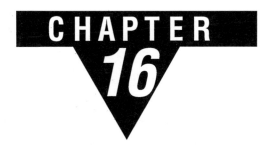

CHAPTER 16

Thorax and Lungs

Purpose: This chapter helps you to learn the structure and function of the thorax and lungs, to understand the methods of examination of the respiratory system, to identify lung sounds that are normal, to describe the characteristics of adventitious lung sounds, and to accurately record the assessment. At the end of this unit you will be able to perform a complete physical examination of the respiratory system.

Reading Assignment: Jarvis, *Physical Examination and Health Assessment*, 2nd ed., Chapter 16, pp.459-511

_____

Audio-Visual Assignment: _____

_____

Glossary: Study the following terms after completing the reading assignment. You should be able to cover the definition on the right and define the term out loud.

Alveoli .... Functional units of the lung; the thin–walled chambers surrounded by networks of capillaries that are the site of respiratory exchange of carbon dioxide and oxygen

Angle of Louis .... Manubriosternal angle, the articulation of the manubrium and body of the sternum, and continuous with the second rib

Apnea .... Cessation of breathing

Asthma .... An abnormal respiratory condition associated with allergic hypersensitivity to certain inhaled allergans, characterized by bronchospasm, wheezing, and dyspnea

Atelectasis .... An abnormal respiratory condition characterized by collapsed, shrunken, deflated section of alveoli

Bradypnea .... Slow breathing, < 10 breaths per minute, regular rate

Bronchiole .... One of the smaller respiratory passageways into which the segmental bronchi divide

Bronchitis .... Inflammation of the bronchi with partial obstruction of bronchi due to excessive mucus secretion

Bronchophony .... The spoken voice sound heard through the stethoscope, which sounds soft, muffled and indistinct over normal lung tissue

Bronchovesicular .... The normal breath sound heard over major bronchi, characterized by moderate pitch and an equal duration of inspiration and expiration

Chronic obstructive
pulmonary disease (COPD) .... A functional category of abnormal respiratory conditions characterized by airflow obstruction, e.g., emphysema, chronic bronchitis

Cilia .... Millions of hair cells lining the tracheobronchial tree

Consolidation .... The solidification of portions of lung tissue as it fills up with infectious exudate, as in pneumonia

Crackles .... (rales) abnormal, discontinuous, adventitious lung sounds heard on inspiration

Crepitus .... Coarse crackling sensation palpable over the skin when air abnormally escapes from the lung and enters the subcutaneous tissue

Dead space .... Passageways that transport air but are not available for gaseous exchange, e.g., trachea and bronchi

Dyspnea .... Difficult, labored breathing

Egophony .... The voice sound of "eeeeee" heard through the stethoscope

Emphysema .... The chronic obstructive pulmonary disease characterized by enlargement of alveoli distal to terminal bronchioles

Fissure .... The narrow crack dividing the lobes of the lungs

Fremitus .... A palpable vibration from the spoken voice felt over the chest wall

Friction rub .... A coarse, grating, adventitious lung sound heard when the pleurae are inflamed

Hypercapnia .... (hypercarbia), increased levels of carbon dioxide in the blood

Hypoxemia .... Decreased level of oxygen in the blood

Hyperventilation .... Increased rate and depth of breathing

Intercostal space .... Space between the ribs

Kussmaul respiration .... A type of hyperventilation that occurs with diabetic ketoacidosis

Orthopnea .... Ability to breath easily only in an upright position

Paroxysmal nocturnal dyspnea . Sudden awakening from sleeping with shortness of breath

Percussion .... Striking over the chest wall with short sharp blows of the fingers in order to determine the size and density of the underlying organ

Pleural effusion .... Abnormal fluid between the layers of the pleura

Rhonchi .... Low pitched, musical, snoring, adventitious lung sound caused by airflow obstruction from secretions

Tachypnea............................... Rapid shallow breathing, > 24 breaths per minute

Vesicular .... The soft, low–pitched, normal breath sound heard over peripheral lung fields

Vital capacity .... The amount of air, following maximal inspiration, that can be exhaled

Wheeze .... High pitched, musical, squeaking adventitious lung sound

Whispered pectoriloquy .... A whispered phrase heard through the stethoscope that sounds faint and inaudible over normal lung tissue

Xiphoid process .... Sword–shaped lower tip of the sternum

STUDY GUIDE

After completing the reading assignment and the audio–visual assignment, you should be able to answer the following questions in the spaces provided.

1. List the questions to obtain a health history for the respiratory system.

2. Describe the pleura and its function.

3. List the structures that comprise the respiratory dead space.

4. Summarize the mechanics of respiration.

5. List the elements included in the inspection of the respiratory system.

6. Discuss the significance of a "barrel chest."

7. List and describe common thoracic deformities.

8. List and describe three (3) types of normal breath sounds.

9. Define two (2) types of adventitious breath sounds.

10. The manubriosternal angle is also called _____.

   Why is is a useful landmark?

11. How many degrees in the normal costal angle? _____

12. When comparing the anterior–posterior diameter of the chest to the transverse diameter, what is the expected ratio?

   What is the significance of this?

13. What is tripod position?

14. List three (3) factors that affect normal intensity of tactile fremitus

    1.

    2.

    3.

15. During percussion, which sound would you expect to predominate over normal lung tissue?

16. Normal findings for diaphragmatic excursion are:

17. List five (5) factors that can cause extraneous noise during auscultation.

    1.

    2.

    3.

    4.

    5.

18. Describe the three (3) types of normal breath sounds:

Name	Location	Description
_____	_____	_____
_____	_____	_____
_____	_____	_____

19. Fill in the labels indicated on the following illustrations

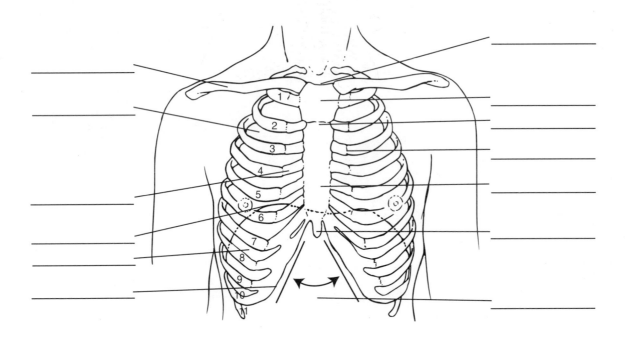

Draw in the lobes of the lungs and label their landmarks on the following two illustrations

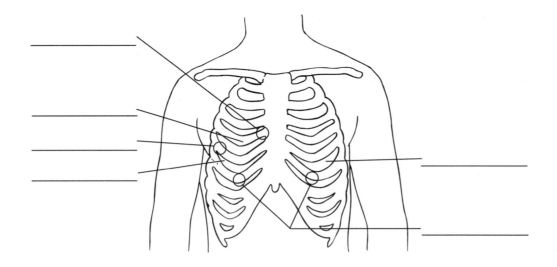

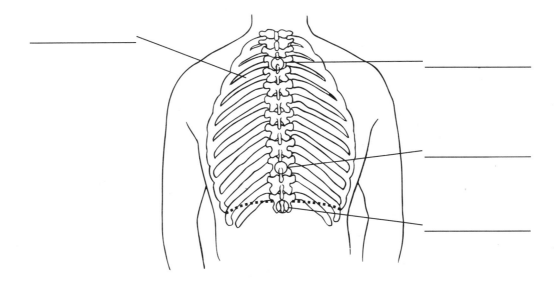

REVIEW QUESTIONS

This test is for you and is intended to check your own mastery of the content. Answers are provided in Appendix A.

1. The manubriosternal angle is:

   a. the articulation of the manubrium and the body of the sternum.
   b. a hollow U-shaped depression just above the sternum.
   c. also know as the breastbone.
   d. a term synonymous with costochondral junction.

2. Select the correct description of the left lung.

   a. narrower than the right lung with three lobes
   b. narrower than the right with two lobes
   c. wider than the right lung with two lobes
   d. shorter than the right with three lobes

3. Some conditions have a cough with characteristic timing. The cough associated with chronic bronchitis is best described as:

   a. continuous throughout the day.
   b. productive cough for three months of the year for 2 years in a row.
   c. occurring in the afternoon/evening because of exposure to irritants at work.
   d. occurring in the early morning.

4. Symmetric chest expansion is best confirmed by:

   a. placing hands on the posterolateral chest wall with thumbs at the level of T9 or T10, then sliding the hands up to pinch up a small fold of skin between the thumbs.

   b. inspection of the shape and configuration of the chest wall.

   c. placing the palmar surface of the fingers of one hand against the chest and having the client repeat the words "ninety-nine".

   d. percussion of the posterior chest.

5. Absence of diaphragmatic excursion occurs with:

   a. asthma.

   b. an unusually thick chest wall.

   c. pleural effusion or atelectasis of the lower lobes.

   d. age related changes in the chest wall.

6. Auscultation of breath sounds is an important component of respiratory assessment. Select the description that most accurately describes this part of the examination.

   a. hold the bell of the stethoscope against the chest wall, listen to the entire right field, then the entire left field.

   b. hold the diaphragm of the stethoscope against the chest wall, listen to one full respiration in each location being sure to do side-to side-comparisons.

   c. listen from the apices to the bases of each lung field using the bell of the stethoscope.

   d. select the bell or diaphragm depending upon the quality of sounds heard, listen for one respiration in each location, moving from side to side.

7. Select the best description of bronchovesicular breath sounds:

   a. high pitched, of longer duration on inspiration than expiration.

   b. moderate pitch, inspiration = to expiration.

   c. low pitched, inspiration greater than expiration.

   d. rustling sound, like the wind in the trees.

8. After examining a client, the practitioner makes the following notation: Increased respiratory rate, chest expansion decreased on left side, dull to percussion over left lower lobe, breath sounds louder with fine crackles over left lower lobe. These findings are consistent with a diagnosis of:

   a. bronchitis

   b. asthma

   c. pleural effusion.

   d. lobar pneumonia

9. Upon examining a client's nails, the practitioner notes that the angle of the nail base is > 160° and the nail base feels spongy to palpation. These findings are consistent with:

   a. adult respiratory distress syndrome.

   b. normal findings for the nails .

   c. chronic, congenital heart disease and COPD.

   d. atelectasis.

10. Upon examination of a client, the practitioner notes a coarse, low pitched sound during both inspiration and expiration. The client complains of pain with breathing. These finding are consistent with:

    a. fine crackles

    b. wheezes

    c. atelectatic crackles

    d. pleural friction rub

11. The practitioner is going to use the technique of egophony. To accomplish this, the client is instructed to:

    a. take several deep breaths, then hold for five seconds.

    b. say "ee" each time the stethoscope is moved.

    c. repeat the phrase "ninety-nine" each time the stethoscope is moved.

    d. whisper a phrase as auscultation is performed.

Match column A to with column B

Column A—lung borders			**Column B—location**
12. ___	apex	a.	rests on the diaphragm
13. ___	base	b.	C7
14. ___	lateral left	c.	sixth rib, midclavicular line
15. ___	lateral right	d.	fifth intercostal space
16. ___	posterior apex	e.	3 - 4 cm above the inner third of the clavicles

Match column A to column B

Column A—configurations of the thorax			**Column B—description**
17. ___	normal chest	a.	anteroposterior = transverse diameter
18. ___	barrel chest	b.	exaggerated posterior curvature of thoracic spine
19. ___	pectus excavatum	c.	lateral S-shaped curvature of the thoracic and lumbar spine
20. ___	pectus carinatum	d.	sunken sternum and adjacent cartilages
21. ___	scoliosis	e.	elliptical shape with an anteroposterior: transverse diameter of 1:2
22. ___	kyphosis	f.	forward protrusion of the sternum with ribs sloping back at either side

SKILLS LABORATORY/ CLINICAL SETTING

Clinical Objectives

You are now ready for the clinical component of the respiratory system. The purpose of the clinical component is to practice the regional examination on a peer in the skills laboratory and to achieve the following.

1. Demonstrate knowledge of the symptoms related to the respiratory system by obtaining a regional health history from a peer/client.

2. Correctly locate anatomic landmarks on the thorax of a peer.

3. Using a grease pencil, and with peer's permission, draw lobes of the lungs on a peer's thorax.

4. Demonstrate correct techniques for inspection, palpation, percussion, and auscultation of the respiratory system.

5. Demonstrate the technique for extimation diaphragmatic excursion.

6. Record the history and physical exam findings accurately, reach an assessment of the health state, amd develop a plan of care.

Instructions

Gather your equipment. Practice the steps of the exam of the thorax and lungs on a peer or on a client in the clinical area. Record your findings using the regional write–up sheet. The front of the sheet is intended as a work sheet, the back of the sheet is intended for a narrative summary using the SOAP format.

REGIONAL WRITE-UP—THORAX AND LUNGS

Date _____

Client _____ Age _____ Sex ___ Occupation _____

Examiner _____

I. Health History

	No	Yes, explain
1. Do you have a **cough**?		
2. Any shortness of **breath**?		
3. Any **chest pain** with breathing?		
4. Any **past history** of lung diseases?		
5. **Smoke** cigarettes? How many/day?		
6. Any living or work conditions that affect your breathing?		
7. Last Tb skin test, chest xray, flu vaccine?		

II. Physical Examination

A. Inspection
1. Thoracic cage _____
2. Respiratory rate and pattern _____
3. Skin _____
4. Person's position _____
5. Facial expression _____
6. Level of consciousness _____

B. Palpation
1. Confirm symmetrical chest expansion _____
2. Tactile fremitus _____
3. Detect any lumps, masses, tenderness _____
4. Trachea _____

C. Percussion
1. Determine percussion note that predominates over lung fields _____
2. Diaphragmatic excursion _____

D. Auscultation
1. Listen: Posterior, Lateral, Anterior _____
2. Any abnormal breath sounds? _____

   If so, perform bronchophony, _____

   whispered pectoriloquy, _____

   egophony _____
3. Any adventitious sounds? _____

REGIONAL WRITE-UP—THORAX AND LUNGS

Summarize your findings using the SOAP format.

Subjective (Client's reason for seeking care, health history)

Objective (Physical exam findings)   Use the drawing to diagram your findings

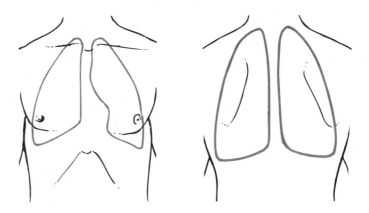

Assessment (Assessment of health state or problem, diagnosis)

Plan (Diagnostic evaluation, follow-up care, teaching)

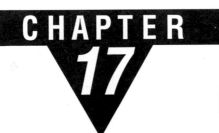

CHAPTER 17

Heart and Neck Vessels

Purpose: This chapter helps you to learn the structure and function of the heart, valves, and great vessels; to understand the cardiac cycle; to describe the heart sounds; to understand the rationale and methods of examination of the heart; and to accurately record the assessment. At the end of this unit you should be able to perform a complete assessment of the heart and neck vessels.

Reading Assignment: Jarvis, *Physical Examination and Health Assessment*, 2nd ed., Chapter 17, pp. 513-567

_____

Audio-Visual Assignment: _____

_____

Glossary: Study the following terms after completing the reading assignment. You should be able to cover the definition on the right and define the term out loud.

Angina pectoris .... acute chest pain that occurs when myocardial demand exceeds its oxygen supply

Aortic regurgitation .... (aortic insufficiency) incompetent aortic valve that allows backward flow of blood into left ventricle during diastole

Aortic stenosis .... calcification of aortic valve cusps that restricts forward flow of blood during systole

Aortic valve .... the left semilunar valve separating the left ventricle and the aorta

Apex of the heart .... tip of the heart pointing down toward the 5th left intercospal space

Apical impulse .... (point of maximal impulse, PMI) pulsation created as the left ventricle rotates against the chest wall during systole, normally at the 5th left intercostal space in the midclavicular line

Base of the heart .... broader area of heart's outline located at the 3rd right and left intercostal space

Bell (of the stethoscope) .... cup-shaped endpiece used for soft, low pitched heart sounds

Bradycardia .... slow heart rate, < 50 beats per minute in the adult

Clubbing .... bulbous enlargement of distal phalanges of fingers and toes that occurs with chronic cyanotic heart and lung conditions

Coarctation of aorta .... severe narrowing of the descending aorta, a congenital heart defect

Cor pulmonale .... right ventricular hypertrophy and heart failure due to pulmonary hypertension

Cyanosis .... dusky blue mottling of the skin and mucous membranes due to excessive amount of reduced hemoglobin in the blood

Diaphragm (of the stethoscope) .. flat endpiece of the stethoscope used for hearing relatively high-pitched heart sounds

Diastole .... the heart's filling phase

Dyspnea .... difficult labored beathing

Edema .... swelling of legs or dependent body part due to increased interstitial fluid

Erb's point .... traditional auscultatory area in the 3rd left intercostal space

First heart sound (S_1) .... occurs with closure of the atrioventricular (AV) valves signaling the beginning of systole

Fourth heart sound (S_4) .... (S_4 gallop, atrial gallop) very soft, low pitched, ventricular filling sound that occurs in late diastole

Gallop rhythm .... the addition of a 3rd or a 4th heart sound makes the rhythm sound like the cadence of a galloping horse

Inching .... technique of moving the stethoscope incrementally across the precordium through the auscultatory areas while listening to the heart sounds

LVH (left ventricular hypertrophy) increase in thickness of myocardial wall that occurs when the heart pumps against chronic outflow obstruction, e.g., aortic stenosis

MCL (midclavicular line) .... imaginary vertical line bisecting the middle of the clavicle in each hemithorax

Mitral regurgitation .... (mitral insufficiency) incompetent mitral valve allows regurgitation of blood back into left atrium during systole

Mitral stenosis .... calcified mitral valve impedes forward flow of blood into left ventricle during diastole

Mitral valve .... left AV valve separating the left atria and ventricle

Palpitation .... uncomfortable awareness of rapid or irregular heartrate

Paradoxical splitting .... opposite of a normal split S_2 so that the split is heard in expiration, and in inspiration the sounds fuse to one sound

Physiologic splitting .... normal variation in S_2 heard as two separate components during inspiration

Precordium .... area of the chest wall overlying the heart and great vessels

Pericardial friction rub .... high-pitched scratchy extracardiac sound heard when the precordium is inflamed

Pulmonary regurgitation .... (pulmonary insufficiency) backflow of blood through incompetent pulmonic valve into the right ventricle

Pulmonary stenosis .... calcification of pulmonic valve that restricts forward flow of blood during systole

Pulmonic valve .... right semilunar valve separating the right ventricle and pulmonary artery

Second heart sound (S_2) .... occurs with closure of the semilunar valves, aortic and pulmonic, and signals the end of systole

Summation gallop .... abnormal mid-diastolic heart sound heard when both the pathologic S_3 and S_4 are present

Syncope .... temporary loss of consciousness due to decreased cerebral blood flow (fainting), caused by ventricular asystole, pronounced brady-cardia, or ventricular fibrillation

Systole .... the heart's pumping phase

Tachycardia .... rapid heart rate, > 100 beats per minute in the adult

Third heart sound (S_3) .... soft, low-pitched, ventricular filling sound that occurs in early diastole (S_3 gallop) and may be an early sign of heart failure

Thrill .... palpable vibration on the chest wall accompanying severe heart murmur

Tricuspid valve .... right AV valve separating the right atria and ventricle

STUDY GUIDE

After completing the reading assignment and the audio-visual assignment, you should be able to answer the following questions in the spaces provided.

1. Define the apical impulse and describe its normal location, size, and duration.

   Which *normal* variations may affect the location of the apical impulse?

   Which *abnormal* conditions may affect the location of the apical impulse?

2. Explain the mechanism producing normal first and second heart sounds.

3 Describe the affect of respiration on the heart sounds.

4. Describe the characteristics of the first heart sound, and its intensity at the apex of the heart and at the base.

Which conditions *increase* the intensity of S_1?

Which conditions *decrease* the intensity of S_1?

5. Describe the characteristics of the second heart sound, and its intensity at the apex of the heart and at the base.

Which conditions *increase* the intensity of S_2?

Which conditions *decrease* the intensity of S_2?

6. Explain the physiologic mechanism for normal splitting of S_2 in the pulmonic valve area.

7. Define the third heart sound. When in the cardiac cycle does it occur? Describe its intensity, quality, location in which it is heard, and method of auscultation.

8. Differentiate a physiologic S_3 from a pathologic S_3.

9. Define the fourth heart sound. When in the cardiac cycle does it occur? Describe its intensity, quality, location in which it is heard, and method of auscultation.

10. Explain the position of the valves during each phase of the cardiac cycle.

11. Define venous pressure and jugular venous pulse.

12. Differentiate between the carotid artery pulsation and the jugular vein pulsation.

13. List the areas of questioning to address during the health history of the cardiovascular system.

14. Define bruit, and discuss what it indicates.

15. Define heave or lift, and discuss what it indicates.

16. State 4 guidelines to distinguish S_1 from S_2.

    1. _____
    2. _____
    3. _____
    4. _____

17. Define pulse deficit and discuss what it indicates.

18. Define preload and afterload.

19. List the characteristics to explore when you hear a murmur, including the grading scale of murmurs.

20. Discuss the characteristics of an innocent or functional murmur.

21. Fill in the labels indicated on the following illustrations.

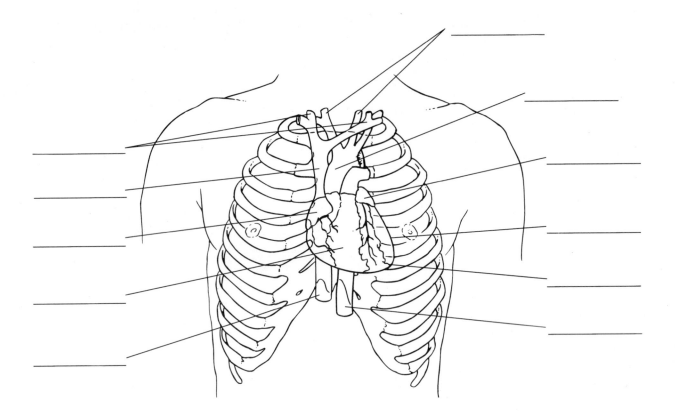

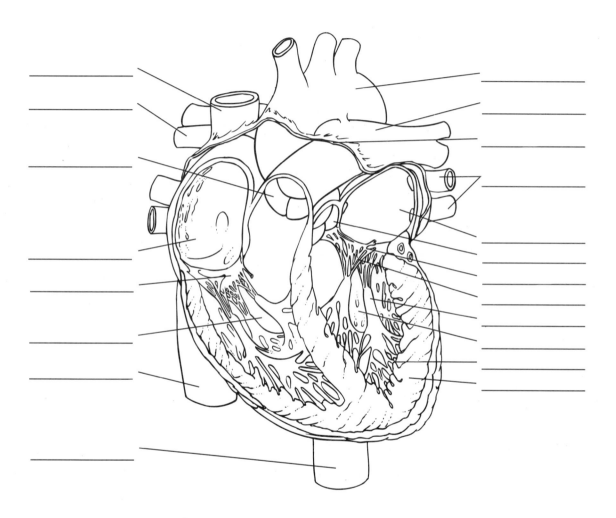

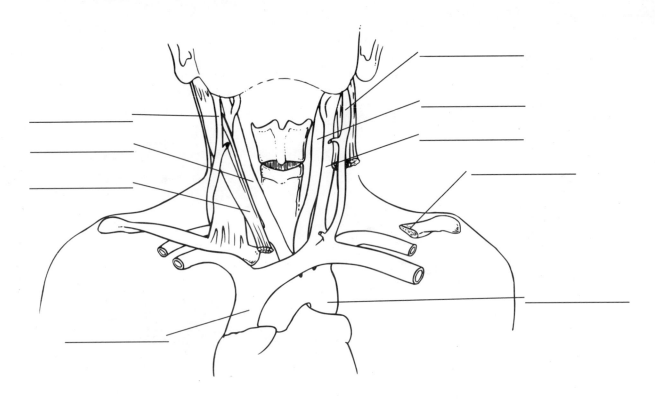

REVIEW QUESTIONS

This test is for you and is intended to check your own mastery of the content. Answers are provided in Appendix A.

1. The precordium is:
   a. a synonym for the mediastinum.
   b. the area on the chest where the apical impulse is felt.
   c. the area on the anterior chest overlying the heart and great vessels.
   d. a synonym for the area where the superior and inferior vena cavae return unoxygenated venous blood to the right side of the heart.

2. Select the best description of the tricuspid valve.
   a. left semilunar valve
   b. right atrioventricular valve
   c. left atrioventricular valve
   d. right semilunar valve.

3. The function of the pulmonic valve is to:
   a. divide the left atrium and left ventricle.
   b. guard the opening between the right atrium and right ventricle.
   c. protect the orifice between the right ventricle and the pulmonary artery.
   d. guard the entrance to the aorta from the left ventricle.

4. Atrial systole occurs:
   a. during ventricular systole.
   b. during ventricular diastole.
   c. concurrently with ventricular systole.
   d. independently of ventricular function.

5. The second heart sound is the result of:

   a.   opening of the mitral and tricuspid valves.
   b.   closing of the mitral and tricuspid valves.
   c.   opening of the aortic and pulmonic valves.
   d.   closing of the aortic and pulmonic valves.

6. The examiner has estimated the jugular venous pressure. Identify the finding that is abnormal .

   a.   Client elevated to 30 degrees, internal jugular vein pulsation at 1 cm above sternal angle.
   b.   Client elevated to 30 degrees, internal jugular vein pulsation at 2 cm above sternal angle.
   c.   Client elevated to 40 degrees, internal jugular vein pulsation at 1 cm above sternal angle.
   d.   Client elevated to 45 degrees, internal jugular vein pulsation at 4 cm above sternal angle.

7. The examiner is palpating the apical impulse. The normal size of this impulse is:

   a.   less than 1 cm.
   b.   about 2 cm.
   c.   3 cm.
   d.   varies depending on the size of the client.

8. The examiner wishes to listen in the pulmonic valve area. To do this, the stethoscope would be placed at the:

   a.   second right interspace.
   b.   second left interspace.
   c.   left lower sternal border.
   d.   fifth interspace, left midclavicular line.

9. Select the statement that best differentiates a split S_2 from S_3.

   a. S_3 is lower pitched and is heard at the apex.
   b. S_2 is heard at the left lower sternal border.
   c.   the timing of S_2 varies with respirations.
   d. S_3 is heard at the base, timing varies with respirations.

10. The examiner wishes to listen for a pericardial friction rub. Select the best method of listening:

   a.   with diaphragm, client sitting up and leaning forward, breath held in expiration
   b.   using the bell with the client leaning forward
   c.   at the base during normal respiration
   d.   with the diaphragm, client turned to the left side

Match column A to to column B

Column A

11. ____   tough, fibrous, double-walled sac that surrounds and protects the heart.

12. ____   thin layer of endothelial tissue that lines the inner surface of the heart chambers and valves

13. ____   reservoir for holding blood

14. ____   ensures smooth friction-free movement of the heart muscle

15. ____   muscular pumping chamber

16. ____   muscular wall of the heart

Column B

   a.   pericardial fluid
   b.   ventricle
   c.   endocardium
   d.   myocardium
   e.   pericardium
   f.   atrium

17. Briefly relate the route of a blood cell from the liver to tissue in the body.

18. List the major risk factors of heart disease and stroke identified in the text.

SKILLS LABORATORY/ CLINICAL SETTING

Clinical Objectives

You are now ready for the clinical component of the cardiovascular system. The purpose of the clinical component is to practice the regional examination on a peer in the skills laboratory and to achieve the following clinical objectives:

1. Demonstrate knowledge of the symptoms related to the cardiovascular system by obtaining a regional health history from a peer or client.

2. Correctly locate anatomic landmarks on the chest wall of a peer.

3. Using a grease pencil, and with peer's permission, outline borders of the heart, and label auscultatory areas on a peer's chest wall.

4. Demonstrate correct technique for inspection and palpation of the neck vessels.

5. Demonstrate correct techniques for inspection, palpation, and auscultation of the percordium.

6. Record the history and physical examination findings accurately, reach an assessment of the health state, and develop a plan of care.

Instructions

Gather your equipment. Practice the steps of the exam of the cardiovascular system on a peer or on a client in the clinical area. Record your findings using the regional write-up sheet that follows. The front of the page is intended as a worksheet; the back of the page is intended for your narrative recording using SOAP format.

REGIONAL WRITE-UP—CARDIOVASCULAR SYSTEM

Date _____

Client _____ Age _____ Sex ___ Occupation _____

Examiner _____

I. Health History

	No	Yes, explain
1. Any **chest pain** or tightness?	_____	_____
2. Any **shortness of breath**?	_____	_____
3. Use more than one pillow to sleep?	_____	_____
4. Do you have a **cough**?	_____	_____
5. Do you seem to **tire easily**?	_____	_____
6. Facial skin ever turn blue or ashen?	_____	_____
7. Any **swelling** of feet or legs?	_____	_____
8. Awaken at night to urinate?	_____	_____
9. Any past history of heart disease?	_____	_____
10. Any family history of heart disease?	_____	_____
11. Assess cardiac risk factors:	_____	_____

II. Physical Examination

A. Carotid Arteries

Inspect and palpate
Grade R _____ L _____
(0 = absent, 1+ weak, 2+ normal, 3+ increased, 4+ bounding)

B. Jugular Venous System

External jugular veins: < collapsed supine
meniscus visible _____

Internal jugular venous pulsations: < not visible
visible at _____

C. Precordium

Inspect and palpate
1. Skin color and condition _____
2. Chest wall pulsations _____
3. Heave or lift _____
4. Apical impulse in the _____ ics at _____
   Size _____ Amplitude _____

D. Auscultation

1. Identify anatomic areas where you will listen.
2. Rate and rhythm _____
3. Identify S_1 and S_2 and note any variation:
   S_1 S_2 S_1 S_2

   S_1 _____
   S_2 _____

4. Listen in systole and diastole:
   Extra heart sounds _____
   Systolic murmur _____
   Diastolic murmur _____

REGIONAL WRITE-UP—CARDIOVASCULAR SYSTEM

Summarize your findings using the SOAP format.

Subjective (Client's reason for seeking care, health history)

Objective (Physical exam findings)   Record findings using diagram

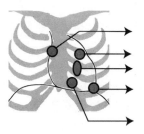

Assessment (Assessment of health state or problem, diagnosis)

Plan (Diagnostic evaluation, follow-up care, client teaching)

CHAPTER 18
Peripheral Vascular System and Lymphatic System

Purpose: This chapter helps you to learn the structure and function of the peripheral vascular system and the lymphatic system; to locate the peripheral pulse sites; to understand the rationale and methods of examination of the peripheral vascular and lymphatic systems; and to accurately record the assessment. At the end of this unit you should be able to perform a complete assessment of the peripheral vascular and lymphatic systems.

Reading Assignment: Jarvis, *Physical Examination and Health Assessment*, 2nd ed., Chapter 18, pp. 569-598

_____

Audio-Visual Assignment: _____

_____

Glossary: Study the following terms after completing the reading assignment. You should be able to cover the definition on the right and define the term out loud.

Allen test	determining the patency of the radial and ulnar arteries by compressing one artery site and observing return of skin color as evidence of patency of the other
Aneurysm	defect or sac formed by dilation in artery wall due to atherosclerosis, trauma, or congenital defect
Arrhythmia	variation from the heart's normal rhythm
Arteriosclerosis	thickening and loss of elasticity of the arterial walls
Atherosclerosis	plaques of fatty deposits form in the inner layer (intima) of the arteries
Bradycardia	slow heart rate, < 50 beats per minute in the adult
Bruit	blowing swooshing sound heard through a stethoscope when an artery is partially occluded
Cyanosis	dusky blue mottling of the skin and mucous membranes due to excessive amount of reduced hemoglobin in the blood
Diastole	the heart's filling phase

Homan's sign .... calf pain that occurs when the foot is sharply dorsiflexed against the calf; may occur with deep vein thrombosis, phlebitis, Achilles tendinitis, or muscle injury

Ischemia .... deficiency of arterial blood to a body part, due to constriction or obstruction of a blood vessel

Lymph nodes .... small oval clumps of lymphatic tissue located at intervals along lymphatic vessels

Lymphedema .... swelling of extremity due to obstructed lymph channel, nonpitting

Pitting edema .... indentation left after examiner depresses the skin over swollen edematous tissue

Profile sign .... viewing the finger from the side in order to detect early clubbing

Pulse .... pressure wave created by each heartbeat, palpable at body sites where the artery lies close to the skin and over a bone

Pulsus alternans .... regular rhythm, but force of pulse varies with alternating beats of large and small amplitude

Pulsus bigeminus .... irregular rhythm, every other beat is premature; premature beats have weakened amplitude

Pulsus paradoxus .... beats have weaker amplitude with respiratory inspiration, stronger with expiration

Systole .... the heart's pumping phase

Tachycardia .... rapid heart rate, > 100 beats per minute in the adult

Thrombophlebitis .... inflammation of the vein associated with thrombus formation

Varicose vein .... dilated tortuous veins with incompetent valves

Ulcer .... open skin lesion extending into dermis with sloughing of necrotic inflammatory tissue

STUDY GUIDE

After completing the reading assignment and the audio-visual assignment, you should be able to answer the following questions in the spaces provided.

1. Describe the structure and function of arteries and veins.

2. List the pulse sites accessible to examination.

3. Describe 3 mechanisms that help return venous blood to the heart.

4. Define capacitance vessels and explain its significance.

5. List the risk factors for venous stasis.

6. Describe the function of the lymphatic system.

7. Describe the function of the lymph nodes.

8. Name the related organs in the lymphatic system.

9. List the symptom areas to address during history taking of the peripheral vascular system.

10. Fill in the grading scale for assessing the force of an arterial pulse: 0 = _____; 1+ _____;

    2+ _____; 3+ _____; 4+ _____

11. List the steps in performing the Allen test.

12. List the skin characteristics expected with arterial insufficiency to the lower legs.

13. Compare the characteristics of leg ulcers associated with arterial insufficiency vs. ulcers with venous insufficiency.

14. Fill in the description of the grading scale for pitting edema:

    1+ _____

    2+ _____

    3+ _____

    4+ _____

15. Describe the technique for using the Doppler Ultrasonic Stethoscope to detect peripheral pulses.

16. Raynaud's syndrome has associated progressive tricolor changes of the skin from _____ to _____ and then to _____. State the mechanism for each of these color changes.

17. Fill in the labels indicated on the following illustration.

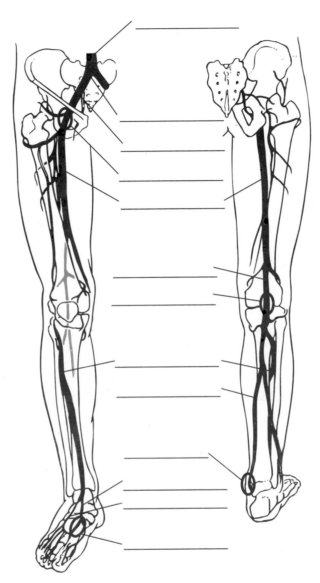

REVIEW QUESTIONS

This test is for you and is intended to check your own mastery of the content. Answers are provided in Appendix A.

1. A function of the venous system is:

    a.   to hold more blood when blood volume increases.

    b.   to conserve fluid and plasma proteins that leak out of the capillaries.

    c.   to form a major part of the immune system that defends the body against disease.

    d.   to absorb lipids from the intestinal tract.

2. The organs that aid the lymphatic system are:

    a.   liver, lymph nodes, and stomach.

    b.   pancreas, small intestines, and thymus.

    c.   spleen, tonsils, and thymus.

    d.   pancreas, spleen, and tonsils.

3. Ms. T. has come for a prenatal visit. She complains of dependent edema, varicosities in the legs, and hemorrhoids. The best response is:

a. "If these symptoms persist, we will perform an amniocentesis."
b. "If these symptoms persist, we will discuss having you hospitalized."
c. "The symptoms are caused by the pressure of the growing uterus on the veins. They are usual conditions of pregnancy."
d. "At this time, the symptoms are a minor inconvenience. We will check again during your next visit."

4. The nurse is checking the pulse of patient who just returned from physical therapy. The pulse has an amplitude of 3+ This would be considered:

a. bounding.
b. increased.
c. normal.
d. weak.

5. Inspection of the client's right hand reveals a red, swollen area. To further assess for infection, the nurse would palpate the:

a. cervical node.
b. the axillary node.
c. the epitrochlear node.
d. the inguinal node.

6. A method for assessing the circulation of the lower extremities is to:

a. measure the circumference of the ankle.
b. check the temperature with the palm of the hand.
c. compress the dorsalis pedis pulse and looking for blood return.
d. measure the widest point with a tape measure.

7. During the examination of the lower extremities, the practitioner is unable to palpate the popliteal pulse. The practitioner should:

a. proceed with the exam. It is often impossible to palpate this pulse.
b. refer the client to a vascular surgeon for further evaluation.
c. schedule the client for a venogram.
d. schedule the client for an arteriogram.

8. While reviewing a medical record, a notation of 4+ edema of the right leg is noted. The best description of this type of edema is:

a. mild pitting, no perceptible swelling of the leg.
b. moderate pitting, indentation subsides rapidly.
c. deep pitting, leg looks swollen.
d. very deep pitting, indentation lasts a long time.

9. The examiner wishes to assess for arterial deficit in the lower extremities. After raising the legs 12 inches off the table and then having the client sit up and dangle the leg the color should return in:

a. 5 seconds or less.
b. 10 seconds or less.
c. 15 seconds.
d. between 10 and 15 seconds.

SKILLS LABORATORY/ CLINICAL SETTING

Clinical Objectives

You are now ready for the clinical component of the peripheral vascular system. The purpose of the clinical component is to practice the regional examination on a peer in the skills laboratory and to achieve the following clinical objectives:

1. Demonstrate knowledge of the symptoms related to the peripheral vascular system by obtaining a regional health history from a peer or client.

2. Demonstrate palpation of peripheral arterial pulses (brachial, radial, femoral, popliteal, posterior tibial, dorsalis pedis) by: assessing amplitude and symmetry; noting any signs of arterial insufficiency.

3. Demonstrate inspection and palpation of peripheral veins by noting any signs of venous insuffficiency.

4. Demonstrate palpation of lymphatic system by identifying enlargement, clumping, or abnormal firmness of regional lymph nodes.

5. Demonstrate correct technique of performing the following additional tests when indicated: Allen test; Trendelenberg test; Manual compression test; Doppler Ultrasonic Stethoscope; computing the Ankle-Arm Index.

6. Record the history and physical examination findings accurately, reach an assessment of the health state, and develop a plan of care.

Instructions

Gather your equipment. Wash your hands. Practice the steps of the exam of the peripheral vascular system on a peer or on a client in the clinical setting, giving appropriate instructions as you proceed. Record your findings using the regional write-up sheets that follow. The first part is intended as a worksheet; the last page is intended for your narrative summary recording using SOAP format. Note that the peripheral examination and cardiovascular examination usually are practiced together.

NOTES

REGIONAL WRITE-UP—PERIPHERAL VASCULAR SYSTEM

Date _____

Client_____ Age _____ Sex ___ Occupation _____

Examiner_____

I. Health History

	No	Yes, explain
1. Any leg **pain** (cramps)? Where?	_____	_____
2. Any **skin changes** in arms or legs?	_____	_____
3. Any sores or **lesions** in arms or legs?	_____	_____
4. Any **swelling** in the legs?	_____	_____
5. Any **swollen glands**? Where?	_____	_____
6. What medications are you taking?	_____	

II. Physical Examination

A. Inspection

1. The Arms

   Inspect

   Color of skin and nailbeds _____

   Symmetry _____

   Lesions _____

   Edema _____

   Clubbing_____

   Palpate

   Temperature _____

   Texture _____

   Capillary refill _____

   Locate and grade pulses (record on back)

   Check epitrochlear lymph node _____

   Allen test (if indicated) _____

2. The Legs

   Inspect

   Color _____

   Hair distribution _____

   Venous pattern/ Varicosities _____

   Size_____

   Swelling/Edema _____

   Atrophy _____

   If so, measure calf circumference in cm R _____ L _____

   Skin lesions or ulcers _____

   Palpate

   Temperature _____

   Check Homan's sign _____

   Tenderness _____

   Inguinal lymph nodes _____

   Locate and grade pulses (record on back)

   Check pretibial edema (grade if present)_____

   Auscultate for bruit (if indicated) _____

	Brachial	Radial	Femoral	Popliteal	D. pedis	P. tibial
R						
L						

0 = absent; 1+ weak; 2+ normal; 3+ full; 4+ bounding

3. Additional Tests

   Manual compression test _____

   Trendelenburg test _____

   Check color change: elevate legs, then dangle, color return in _____ seconds

   Doppler Ultrasonic Stethoscope

      Locate pulse sites

      Ankle-Arm Index (AAI)

         _____ ankle systolic pressure

   $$\overline{\hspace{6cm}} \quad = \_.\_\_\_\_ \text{ or } \_\_\_\_ \%$$

         _____ arm systolic pressure

REGIONAL WRITE-UP—PERIPHERAL VASCULAR SYSTEM

Summarize your findings using the SOAP format.

Subjective (Client's reason for seeking care, health history)

Objective (Physical exam findings)   (Record the pulses on the diagram below)

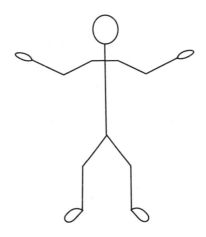

Assessment (Assessment of health state or problem, diagnosis)

Plan (Diagnostic evaluation, follow-up care, client teaching)

CHAPTER 19

Abdomen

Purpose: This chapter helps you to learn the structure and function of the abdominal organs; to know the location of the abdominal organs; to discriminate normal bowel sounds; to understand the rationale and methods of examination of the abdomen; and to accurately record the assessment. At the end of this chapter you should be able to perform a complete assessment of the abdomen.

Reading Assignment: Jarvis, *Physical Examination and Health Assessment*, 2nd ed., Chapter 19, pp. 599-643

Audio-Visual Assignment: _____

_____

Glossary: Study the following terms after completing the reading assignment. You should be able to cover the definition on the right and define the term out loud.

Aneurysm .... defect or sac formed by dilation in artery wall due to atherosclerosis, trauma, or congenital defect

Anorexia .... loss of appetite for food

Ascites .... abnormal accumulation of serous fluid within the peritoneal cavity, associated with congestive heart failure, cirrhosis, cancer, or portal hypertension

Borborygmi .... loud gurgling bowel sounds signaling increased motility or hyperperistalsis, occur with early bowel obstruction, gastroenteritis, diarrhea

Bruit .... blowing swooshing sound heard through a stethoscope when an artery is partially occluded

Cecum .... first or proximal part of large intestine

Cholecystitis .... inflammation of the gallbladder

Costal margin .... lower border of rib margin formed by the medial edges of the 8th, 9th, 10th ribs

Costovertebral angle (CVA)..... angle formed by the 12th rib and the vertebral column on the posterior thorax, overlying the kidney

Diastasis recti .... midline longitudinal ridge in the abdomen, a separation of abdominal rectus muscles

Dysphagia .... difficulty swallowing

Epigastrium .... name of abdominal region between the costal margins

Hepatomegaly .... abnormal enlargement of liver

Hernia   .... abnormal protrusion of bowel through weakening in abdominal musculature

Inguinal ligament..................... ligament extending from pubic bone to anterior superior iliac spine, forming lower border of abdomen

Linea alba .... midline tendinous seam joining the abdominal muscles

Paralytic ileus .... complete absence of peristaltic movement that may follow abdominal surgery or complete bowel obstruction

Peritoneal friction rub.............. rough grating sound heard through the stethoscope over the site of peritoneal inflammation

Peritonitis .... inflammation of peritoneum

Pyloric stenosis .... congenital narrowing of pyloric sphincter, forming outflow obstruction of stomach

Pyrosis   .... (heartburn) burning sensation in upper abdomen, due to reflux of gastric acid

Rectus abdominis muscle .... midline abdominal muscles extending from rib cage to pubic bone

Scaphoid   .... abnormally sunken abdominal wall as with malnutrition or underweight

Splenomegaly .... abnormal enlargement of spleen

Striae   .... (linea albicantes) silvery white or pink scar tissue formed by stretching of abdominal skin as with pregnancy or obesity

Suprapubic .... name of abdominal region just superior to pubic bone

Tympany   .... high-pitched, musical, drumlike percussion note heard when percussing over the stomach and intestine

Umbilicus .... depression on the abdomen marking site of entry of umbilical cord

Viscera   .... internal organs

STUDY GUIDE

After completing the reading assignment and the audio-visual assignment, you should be able to answer the following questions in the spaces provided.

1. Draw a picture of the abdomen and label its contents.

2. Name the organs that are normally palpable in the abdomen.

3. Describe the proper positioning and preparation of the client for the exam.

4. State the rationale for performing auscultation of the abdomen before palpation or percussion.

5. Discuss inspection of the abdomen, including findings that should be noted.

6. Describe the procedure for auscultation of bowel sounds.

7. Differentiate the following abdominal sounds: normal, hyperactive and hypoactive bowel sounds, succession splash, bruit.

8. Identify and give the rationale for each of the percussion notes heard over the abodmen.

List 4 conditions that may alter normal percussion notes.

9. Describe the procedure for percussing the liver span and the spleen.

10. Describe these maneuvers and discuss their significance: fluid wave test, shifting dullness.

11. Differentiate between light and deep palpation and explain the purpose of each.

List two abnormalities that may be detected by light palpation and two detected by deep palpation.

12. Contrast rigidity with voluntary guarding.

13. Contrast visceral pain and somatic (parietal) pain.

14. Describe rebound tenderness.

15. Describe palpation of the liver, spleen, kidney.

16. Distinguish abdominal wall masses from intra-abdominal masses.

17. Describe the procedure and rationale for determining costovertebral angle (CVA) tenderness.

18. Describe the expected examination findings of the abdomen in each of the following conditions:

Obesity _____

Gaseous distention _____

Tumor _____

Pregnancy _____

Ascites _____

Enlarged liver _____

Enlarged spleen _____

Distended bladder _____

Appendicitis _____

19. Fill in the labels indicated on the folllowing illustrations.

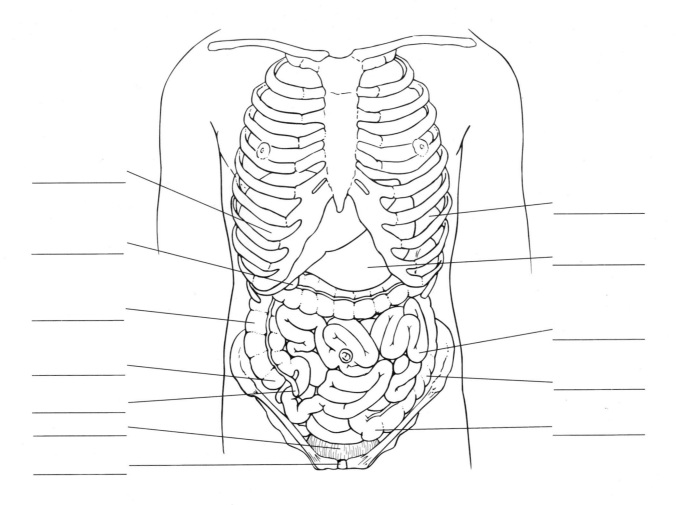

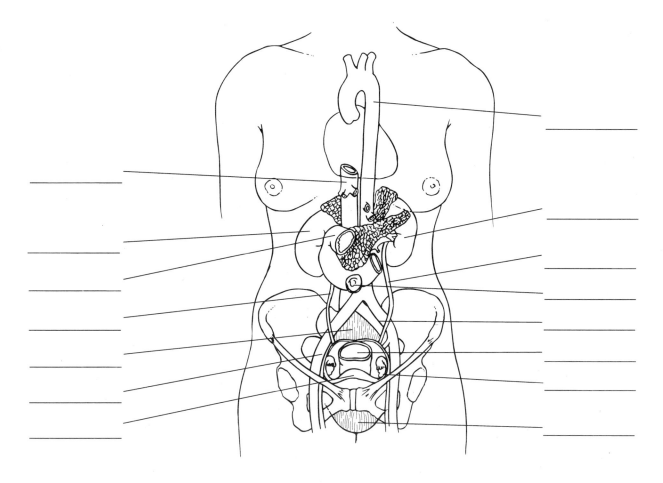

REVIEW QUESTIONS

This test is for you and is intended to check your own mastery of the content. Answers are provided in Appendix A.

1. Select the sequence of techniques used during an examination of the abdomen.

   a. percussion, inspection, palpation, auscultation

   b. inspection, palpation, percussion, auscultation

   c. inspection, auscultation, percussion, palpation

   d. auscultation, inspection, palpation, percussion

2. Which of the following may be noted through inspection of the abdomen?

   a. peristaltic waves and abdominal contour

   b. abdominal contour only

   c. venous pattern, peristaltic waves and abdominal contour

   d. peritoneal irritation, venous patterns and peristaltic waves

3. Right upper quadrant tenderness may indicate pathology in the:

    a.   liver, pancreas, and ascending colon.
    b.   liver and stomach.
    c.   sigmoid colon, spleen and rectum.
    d.   appendix and ileocecal valve.

4. Borborygmi, or hyperactive bowel sounds are:

    a.   high-pitched.
    b.   rushing.
    c.   tinkling.
    d.   all of the above.

5. The absence of bowel sounds is established after listening for:

    a.   1 full minute.
    b   3 full minutes.
    c.   5 full minutes.
    d.   none of the above.

6. Auscultation of the abdomen may reveal bruits of the ___arteries.

    a.   aortic, renal, iliac, and femoral
    b.   jugular, aortic, carotid, and femoral
    c.   pulmonic, aortic, and portal
    d.   renal, iliac, internal jugular, and basilic

7. The size of the liver is determined through percussion. The span of a normal adult liver is:

    a.   7 - 11 cm.
    b.   4 - 8 cm.
    c.   5 - 10 cm.
    d.   6 - 12 cm.

8. The left upper quadrant (LUQ) contains the:

    a.   liver.
    b.   appendix.
    c.   left ovary.
    d.   spleen.

9. Striae, which occur when the elastic fibers in the reticular layer of the skin are broken following rapid or prolonged stretching, have a distinct color when of long duration. This color is:

    a.   pink.
    b.   blue.
    c.   purple-blue.
    d.   silvery white.

10. Auscultation of the abdomen is begun in the Right Lower Quadrant (RLQ) because:

    a.   bowel sounds are normally present here.
    b.   peristalsis through the ascending colon is usually active.
    c.   digestion of food causes an increase in peristaltic waves.
    d.   vascular sounds are best heard in this area.

11. A dull percussion note forward of the left midaxillary line is:

    a.   normal, an expected finding during splenic percussion.
    b.   expected between the 8th and 12th ribs.
    c.   found if the exam follows a large meal.
    d.   indicates splenic enlargement.

12. Shifting dullness is a test for:

    a.   ascites.
    b.   splenic enlargement.
    c.   inflammation of the kidney.
    d.   hepatomegaly.

13. Tenderness during abdominal palpation is expected when palpating:

    a.   the liver edge.
    b.   the spleen
    c.   the sigmoid colon
    d.   the kidneys.

14. Murphy's sign is best described as:

    a.   the pain felt when the hand of the examiner is rapidly removed from an inflamed appendix.
    b.   pain felt when taking a deep breath when the examiners fingers are on the approximate location of the gallbladder.
    c.   a sharp pain felt by the client when one hand of the examiner is used to thump the other at the costovertebral angle
    d.   not a valid examination technique.

SKILLS LABORATORY/ CLINICAL SETTING

Clinical Objectives

You are now ready for the clinical component of the abdominal system. The purpose of the clinical component is to practice the regional examination on a peer in the skills laboratory and to achieve the following clinical objectives:

1. Demonstrate knowledge of the symptoms related to the abdominal system by obtaining a regional health history from a peer or client.

2. Demonstrate inspection of the abdomen by assessing skin condition, symmetry, contour, pulsation, umbilicus, nutritional state.

3. Demonstrate auscultation of the abdomen by assessing characteristics of bowel sounds and by screening for bruits.

4. Demonstrate percussion of the abdomen by: identifying predominent percussion note; determining liver span; noting borders of spleen.

5. Demonstrate light palpation by assessing muscular resistance, tenderness, any masses.

6. Demonstrate deep palpation by assessing for: any masses; the liver, spleen, kidneys, aorta; any CVA or rebound tenderness.

7. Demonstrate correct technique of performing the following additional tests when indicated: inspiratory arrest; iliopsoas muscle test; obturator test.

8. Record the history and physical examination findings accurately, reach an assessment of the health state, and develop a plan of care.

Instructions

Gather your equipment. Wash your hands. Assess the client's comfort before starting. Practice the steps of the exam on a peer or a client in the clinical setting, giving appropriate instructions as you proceed. Record your findings using the regional write-up sheets that follow. The front of the page is intended as a worksheet; the back of the page is intended for your narrative summary recording using the SOAP format.

NOTES

REGIONAL WRITE-UP—ABDOMEN

Date _____

Client _____ Age _____ Sex ____ Occupation _____

Examiner _____

I. Health History

		No	Yes, explain

1. Any change in **appetite**? Loss? _____
2. Any difficulty **swallowing**? _____
3. Any foods you cannot tolerate? _____
4. Any **abdominal pain**? _____
5. Any **nausea** or **vomiting**? _____
6. How often are bowel movements? _____
7. Any past history of GI disease? _____
8. What medications are you taking? _____
9. Tell me all food you ate last 24 hours, starting with:
    breakfast   snack   lunch   snack   dinner   snack

II. Physical Examination

A. Inspection
Contour of abdomen _____
General symmetry _____
Skin color and condition _____
Pulsation or movement _____
Umbilicus _____
Hair distribution _____
State of hydration and nutrition _____
Person's facial expression and position in bed _____

B. Auscultation
Bowel sounds _____
Note any vascular sounds _____

C. Percussion
Percuss in all 4 quadrants _____
Percuss borders of liver span in R MCL _____ cm
Percuss spleen _____
If suspect ascites, test for fluid wave and shifting dullness _____

D. Palpation
Light palpation in all 4 quadrants
    Muscle wall _____
    Tenderness _____
    Enlarged organs _____
    Masses _____
Deep palpation in all 4 quadrants
    Masses _____
    Contour of liver _____
    Spleen _____
    Kidneys _____
    Aorta _____
    Rebound tenderness _____
    CVA tenderness _____

E. Additional tests, if indicated

REGIONAL WRITE-UP—ABDOMEN

Summarize your findings using the SOAP format.

Subjective (Client's reason for seeking care, health history)

Objective (Physical exam findings)   (Record findings on diagram)

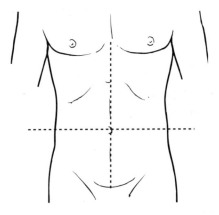

Assessment (Assessment of health state or problem, diagnosis)

Plan (Diagnostic evaluation, follow-up care, client teaching)

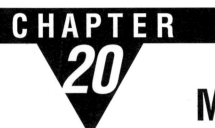

CHAPTER 20

Musculoskeletal System

Purpose: This chapter helps you to learn the structure and function of the various joints in the body; to know their normal ranges of motion; to position the client comfortably during the examination; to understand the rationale and methods of examination of the musculoskeletal system; to assess functional ability; and to accurately record the assessment. At the end of this unit you should be able to perform a complete assessment of the musculoskeletal system.

Reading Assignment: Jarvis, *Physical Examination and Health Assessment*, 2nd ed., Chapter 20, pp. 645-708

_____

Audio-Visual Assignment: _____

_____

Glossary: Study the following terms after completing the reading assignment. You should be able to cover the definition on the right and define the term out loud.

Abduction .... moving a body part away from an axis or the median line

Adduction .... moving a body part toward the center or toward the median line

Ankylosis .... immobility, consolidation, and fixation of a joint because of disease, injury, or surgery; most often due to chronic rheumatoid arthritis

Ataxia .... inability to perform coordinated movements

Bursa .... enclosed sac filled with viscous fluid located in joint areas of potential friction

Circumduction .... moving the arm in a circle around the shoulder

Crepitation .... dry crackling sound or sensation due to grating of the ends of damaged bone

Dorsa .... directed toward or located on the surface

Dupuytren's contracture............ flexion contractures of the fingers due to chronic hyperplasia of the palmar fascia

Eversion .... moving the sole of the foot outward at the ankle

Extension .... straightening a limb at a joint

Flexion	bending a limb at a joint
Ganglion	round, cystic, nontender nodule overlying a tendon sheath or joint capsule, usually on dorsum of wrist
Hallux valgus	lateral or outward deviation of the toe
Inversion	moving the sole of the foot inward at the ankle
Kyphosis	outward or convex curvature of the thoracic spine, hunchback
Ligament	fibrous bands running directly from one bone to another bone that strengthen the joint
Lordosis	inward or concave curvature of the lumbar spine
Nucleus pulposus	center of the intervertebral disc
Olecranon precess	bony projection of the ulna at the elbow
Patella	kneecap
Plantar	surface of the sole of the foot
Pronation	turning the forearm so that the palm is down
Protraction	moving a body part forward and parallel to the gound
Range of motion (ROM)	extent of movement of a joint
Retraction	moving a body part backward and parallel to the gound
Rhematoid arthritis	chronic systemic inflammatory disease of joints and surrounding connective tissue
Sciatica	nerve pain along the course of the sciatic nerve that travels down from the back or thigh through the leg and into the foot
Scoliosis	S-shaped curvature of the thoracic spine
Supination	turning the forearm so that the palm is up
Talipes equinovarus	(clubfoot) congenital deformity of the foot in which it is plantar flexed and inverted
Tendon	strong fibrous cord that attaches a skeletal muscle to a bone
Torticollis	(wryneck) contraction of the cervical neck muscles, producing torsion of the neck

STUDY GUIDE

After completing the reading assignment and the audio-visual assignment, you should be able to answer the following questions in the spaces provided.

1. List 4 signs that suggest acute inflammation in a joint.

2. Differentiate the following:

   dislocation

   subluxation

   contracture

   ankylosis

3. Describe the correct method for use of the goniometer.

4. Differentiate testing of active range of motion vs. passive range of motion.

5. State the expected range of degrees of flexion and extension of the following joints:

   elbow

   wrist

   fingers (at metacarpophalangeal joints)

6. State the expected range of degrees of flexion and extension of the following joints:

   hip

   knee

   ankle

7. Explain the method for measuring leg length.

8. Describe the Ortolani maneuver for checking an infant's hips.

9. State 4 landmarks to note when checking an adolescent for scoliosis.

10. When performing a functional assessment for an older adult, state the common adaptations the aging person makes when attempting these maneuvers:

   Walking _____

   Climbing up stairs _____

   Walking down stairs _____

   Picking up object from floor _____

   Rising up from sitting in chair _____

   Rising up from lying in bed _____

11. Describe the symptoms and signs in carpal tunnel syndrome.

   Name and describe two techniques of examination for the syndrome.

12. Draw and describe Swan-neck deformity and Boutonniere deformity.

13. Contrast Bouchard's nodes from Heberden's nodes.

14. Contrast syndactyly and polydactyly.

15.   Fill in the labels indicated on the following illustrations.

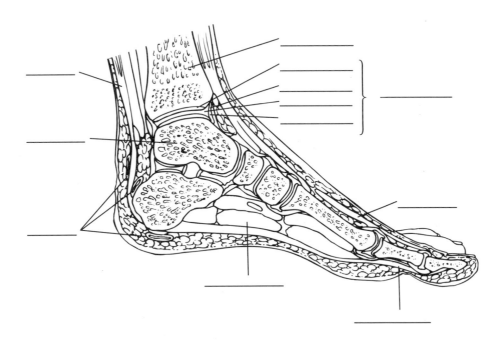

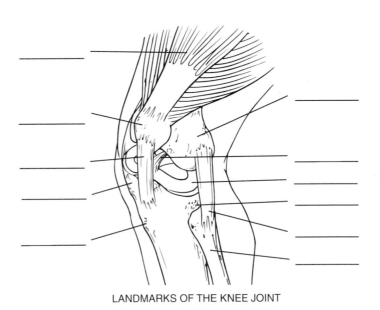

LANDMARKS OF THE KNEE JOINT

REVIEW QUESTIONS

This test is for you and is intended to check your own mastery of the content. Answers are provided in Appendix A.

1. During an assessment of the spine, the client would asked be to:

   a.   adduct, and extend.
   b.   supinate, evert and retract.
   c.   extend, adduct, invert and rotate.
   d.   flex, extend, abduct and rotate.

2. Pronation and supination of the hand and forearm are the result of the articulation of the:

   a.   scapula and clavicle.
   b.   radius and ulna.
   c.   patella and condyle of fibula.
   d.   femur and acetabulum.

3. Anterior and posterior stability is provided to the knee joint by the:

   a.   medial and lateral menisci.
   b.   patellar tendon and ligament.
   c.   medial collateral ligament and quadriceps muscle.
   d.   anterior and posterior cruciate ligaments.

4. A 70-year-old client has come for a health exam. Which of the following is a normal age related change in the curvature of the spinal column.?

   a.   Lordosis
   b.   Scoliosis
   c.   Kyphosis
   d.   Lateral scoliosis

5. The timing of joint pain may assist the examiner in determining the cause. The joint pain associated with rheumatic fever would:

   a.   be worse in the morning.
   b.   be worse later in the day.
   c.   be worse in the morning but improve during the day.
   d.   occur 10 to 14 days after a sore throat.

6. Examination of the shoulder includes four motions. These are:

   a.   forward flexion, internal rotation, abduction, and external rotation.
   b.   abduction, adduction, pronation, and supination.
   c.   circumduction, inversion, eversion, and rotation.
   d.   elevation, retraction, protraction, and circumduction.

7. The Bulge Sign is a test for:

   a.   swelling in the suprapatellar pouch.
   b.   carpal tunnel syndrome.
   c.   Heberden's nodules.
   d.   olecranon bursa inflammation.

8. The examiner is going to measure the client's legs for length discrepancy. The normal finding would be:

   a.   no difference in measurements.
   b.   0.5 or greater.
   c.   within 1 cm of each other.
   d.   2 cm or less.

9. A 2-year-old child has been brought to the clinic for a health examination. A normal finding would be:

   a.   Kyphosis.
   b.   Lordosis.
   c.   Scoliosis.
   d.   No deviation is normal.

10. Briefly describe the functions of the musculoskeletal system.

Match column A with column B

Column A—Movement

11. ____ Flexion

12. ____ Extension

13. ____ Abduction

14. ____ Adduction

15. ____ Pronation

16. ____ Supination

17. ____ Circumduction

18. ____ Inversion

19. ____ Eversion

20. ____ Rotation

21. ____ Protraction

22. ____ Retraction

23. ____ Elevation

24. ____ Depression

Column B—description

a. turning the forearm so that the palm is up

b. binding a limb at a joint

c. lowering a body part

d. turning the forearm so that the palm is down

e. straightening a limb at a joint

f. raising a body part

g. moving a limb away from the midline of the body

h. moving a body part backward and parallel to the ground

i. moving a limb toward the midline of the body

j. moving the arm in a circle around the shoulder

k. moving the sole of the foot outward at the ankle

l. moving a body part forward and parallel to the ground

m. moving the sole of the foot inward at the ankle

n. moving the head around a central axis

SKILLS LABORATORY/ CLINICAL SETTING
Clinical Objectives

You are now ready for the clinical component of the musculoskeletal system. The purpose of the clinical component is to practice the regional examination on a peer in the skills laboratory and to achieve the following clinical objectives:

1. Demonstrate knowledge of the symptoms related to the musculoskeletal system by obtaining a regional health history from a peer or client.

2. Demonstrate inspection and palpation of the musculoskeletal system by assessing the muscles, bones, and joints for: size, symmetry, swelling, nodules, deformities, atrophy, active range of motion.

3. Assess the person's ability to carry out functional activities of daily living.

4. Record the history and physical examination findings accurately, reach an assessment about the health state, and develop a plan of care..

Instructions

Gather your equipment. Wash your hands. Practice the steps of the exam on a peer or a client in the clinical setting, giving appropriate instructions as you proceed, and maintaining the safety of the person during movement. Record your findings using the regional write-up sheet that follows. The first section is intended as a worksheet; the last page is intended for your narrative summary recording using the SOAP format.

REGIONAL WRITE-UP—MUSCULOSKELETAL SYSTEM

Date _____

Client_____ Age_____ Sex___ Occupation_____

Examiner_____

I. Health History

		No	Yes, explain
1.	Any **pain** in the joints?		
2.	Any **stiffness** in the joints?		
3.	Any **swelling, heat, redness** in joints?		
4.	Any **limitation of movement**?		
5.	Any **muscle pain** or cramping?		
6.	Any **deformity** of bone or joint?		
7.	Any **accidents or trauma** to bones?		
8.	Ever had **back pain**?		
9.	Any problems with the activities of daily living:? bathing, toileting, dressing, grooming, eating, mobility, communicating?		

II. Physical Examination

A. Cervical Spine

1. Inspect size and contour
   Color, swelling
   Mass or deformity
2. Palpate for temperature
   Pain
   Swelling or mass
3. Active Range of motion
   Flexion_____ Extension_____
   Lateral bending Right_____ Left_____
   Rotation Right_____ Left_____

B. Shoulders

1. Inspect size and contour
   Color, swelling
   Mass or deformity
2. Palpate for temperature
   Pain
   Swelling or mass
3. Active range of motion
   Flexion_____ Extension_____
   Abduction_____ Adduction_____
   Internal rotation_____ External rotation_____

C. Elbows
1. Inspect for size and contour
    Color, swelling
    Mass or deformity
2. Palpate for temperature
    Pain
    Swelling or mass
3. Active range of motion
    Flexion _____ Extension _____
    Pronation _____ Supination _____

D. Wrists and hands
1. Inspect for size and contour
    Color, swelling
    Mass or deformity
2. Palpate for temperature
    Pain
    Swelling or mass
3. Active range of motion
    Wrist extension _____ Flexion _____
    Finger extension _____ Flexion _____
    Ulnar deviation _____ Radial deviation _____
    Fingers spread _____ Make fist _____
    Touch thumb to each finger _____

E. Hips
1. Inspect for size and contour
    Color, swelling
    Mass or deformity
2. Palpate for temperature
    Pain
    Swelling or mass
3. Active range of motion
    Extension _____ Flexion _____
    External rotation _____ Internal rotation _____
    Abduction _____ Adduction _____

F. Knees
1. Inspect for size and contour
    Color, swelling
    Mass or deformity
2. Palpate for temperature
    Pain
    Swelling or mass
3. Active range of motion
    Flexion _____ Extension _____
    Walk _____ Shallow knee bend _____

G. Ankles and Feet
1. Inspect for size and contour
   Color, swelling
   Mass or deformity
2. Palpate for temperature
   Pain
   Swelling or mass
3. Active range of motion
   Dorsiflexion _____ Plantar flexion _____
   .Inversion _____ Eversion _____

H. Spine
1. Inspect for straight spinous processes
   Equal horizontal positions for: shoulders, scapulae, iliac crests, gluteal folds
   Equal spaces between arm and lateral thorax
   Knees and feet align with trunk, point forward
   From side note curvature: cervical, thoracic, lumbar
2. Palpate spinous processes
3. Active range of motion
   Flexion_____ Extension_____
   Lateral bending right_____ Left_____
   Rotation right _____ Left _____

I. Additional tests (if indicated)
Phalen's test
Tinel's sign
Bulge sign
Ballottement
McMurray's test
Straight leg raising
Measure leg length discrepancy

J. Functional Assessment (if indicated)
Walk (with shoes on)
Climb up stairs
Walk down stairs
Pick up object from floor
Rise up from sitting in chair
Rise up from lying in bed

REGIONAL WRITE-UP—MUSCULOSKELETAL SYSTEM

Summarize your findings using the SOAP format.

Subjective (Client's reason for seeking care, health history)

Objective (Physical exam findings)

Assessment (Assessment of health state or problem, diagnosis)

Plan (Diagnostic evaluation, follow-up care, client teaching)

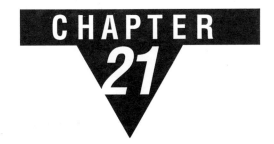

CHAPTER 21

Neurologic System

Purpose: This chapter helps you to learn the structure and function of the components of the neurologic system including the cranial nerves, cerebellar system, motor system, sensory system, and reflexes; to understand the rationale and methods of examination of the neurologic system; and to accurately record the assessment. Together with the mental status assessment presented in Chapter 6, at the end of this unit you should be able to perform a complete assessment of the neurologic system.

Reading Assignment: Jarvis, *Physical Examination and Health Assessment*, 2nd ed., Chapter 21, pp. 709-772

_____

Audio-Visual Assignment: _____

_____

Glossary: Study the following terms after completing the reading assignment. You should be able to cover the definition on the right and define the term out loud.

Agnosia	loss of ability to recognize importance of sensory impressions
Agraphia	loss of ability to express thoughts in writing
Amnesia	loss of memory
Analgesia	loss of pain sensation
Aphasia	loss of power of expression by speech, writing, or signs, or of comprehension of spoken or written language
Apraxia	loss of ability to perform purposeful movements in the absence of sensory or motor damage, e.g., inability to use objects correctly
Ataxia	inability to perform coordinated movements
Athetosis	bizarre, slow, twisting, writhing movement, resembling a snake or worm
Chorea	sudden, rapid, jerky, purposeless movement involving limbs, trunk, or face

Clonus .... rapidly alternating involuntary contraction and relaxation of a muscle in response to sudden stretch

Coma .... state of profound unconsciousness from which person cannot be aroused

Decerebrate rigidity .... arms stiffly extended, adducted, internally rotated; legs stiffly extended, plantar flexed

Decorticate rigidity .... arms adducted and flexed, wrists and fingers flexed; legs extended, internally rotated, plantar flexed

Dysarthria .... imperfect articulation of speech due to problems of muscular control resulting from central or peripheral nervous system damage

Dysphasia .... impairment in speech consisting of lack of coordination and inability to arrange words in their proper order

Extinction .... disappearance of conditioned response

Fasciculation .... rapid continuous twitching of resting muscle without movement of limb

Flaccidity .... loss of muscle tone, limp

Graphesthesia .... ability to "read" a number by having it traced on the skin

Hemiplegia .... loss of motor power (paralysis) on one side of the body, usually caused by a cerebral vascular accident; paralysis occurs on the side opposite the lesion

Lower motor neuron .... motor neuron in the peripheral nervous system with its nerve fiber extending out to the muscle and only its cell body in the central nervous system

Myoclonus .... rapid sudden jerk of a muscle

Nuchal rigidity .... stiffness in cervical neck area

Nystagmus .... back-and-forth oscillation of the eyes

Opisthotonos .... prolonged arching of back, with head and heels bent backward, and meningeal irritation

Paralysis .... decreased or loss of motor function due to problem with motor nerve or muscle fibers

Paraplegia .... impairment or loss of motor and/or sensory function in the lower half of the body

Paresthesia .... abnormal sensation, i.e., burning, numbness, tingling, prickling, crawling skin senstion

Point localization .... ability of the person to discriminate exactly where on the body the skin has been touched

Proprioception .... sensory information concerning body movements and position of the body in space

Spasticity .... continuous resistance to stretching by a muscle due to abnormally increased tension, with increased deep tendon reflexes

Stereognosis........................... ability to recognize objects by feeling their forms, sizes, and weights while the eyes are closed

Tic .... repetitive twitching of a muscle group at inappropriate times, e.g., wink, grimace

Tremor .... involuntary contraction of opposing muscle groups resulting in rhythmic movement of one or more joints

Two-point discrimination .... ability to distinguish the separation of two simultaneous pin pricks on the skin

Upper motor neuron .... nerve located entirely within the central nervous system

STUDY GUIDE

After completing the reading assignment and the audio-visual assignment, you should be able to answer the following questions in the spaces provided.

1. List the major function(s) of the following components of the central nervous system:

   cerebral cortex—frontal lobe _____

   cerebral cortex—parietal lobe _____

   cerebral cortex—temporal lobe _____

   cerebral cortex—Wernicke's area _____

   cerebral cortex—Broca's area _____

   Basal ganglia _____

   Thalamus _____

   Hypothalamus _____

   Cerebellum _____

   Midbrain _____

   Pons _____

   Medulla _____

   Spinal cord _____

2. List the primary sensations mediated by the two major sensory pathways of the CNS.

3. Describe 3 major motor pathways in the CNS including the type of movements mediated by each.

4. Differentiate an upper motor neuron from a lower motor neuron.

5. List the 5 components of a deep tendon reflex arc.

6. List the major symptom areas to assess when collecting a health history for the neurologic system.

7. List the method of testing for each of the 12 cranial nerves.

8. List and describe 3 tests of cerebellar function.

9. Describe the method of testing the sensory system for pain, temperature, touch, vibration, and position.

10. Define the 4 point grading scale for deep tendon reflexes.

11. State the vertebral level whose intactness is assessed when eliciting each of these reflexes:

    biceps reflex_____

    triceps reflex_____

    brachioradialis reflex_____

    quadriceps reflex _____

    achilles reflex _____

12. List the components of the neurologic recheck examination that are performed routinely on hospitalized persons being monitored for neurologic deficit.

13. List the 3 areas of assessment on the Glasgow Coma Scale.

14. Describe the gait patterns of the following abnormal gaits:

    spastic hemiparesis

    cerebellar ataxia

    parkinsonian

    scissors

    steppage

    waddling

15. State the type of reflex response you would expect to see with an upper motor neuron lesion vs. a lower motor neuron lesion.

16. Describe the method of testing the type of reflexes that are also termed frontal release signs.

17. Fill in the labels indicated on the following illustrations.

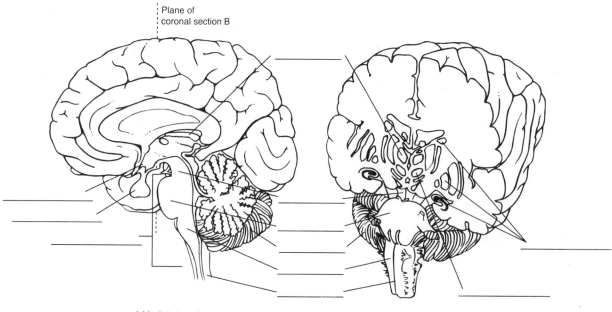

Plane of
coronal section B

A Medial view of right hemisphere

B Coronal section

COMPONENTS OF THE CENTRAL; NERVOUS SYSTEM

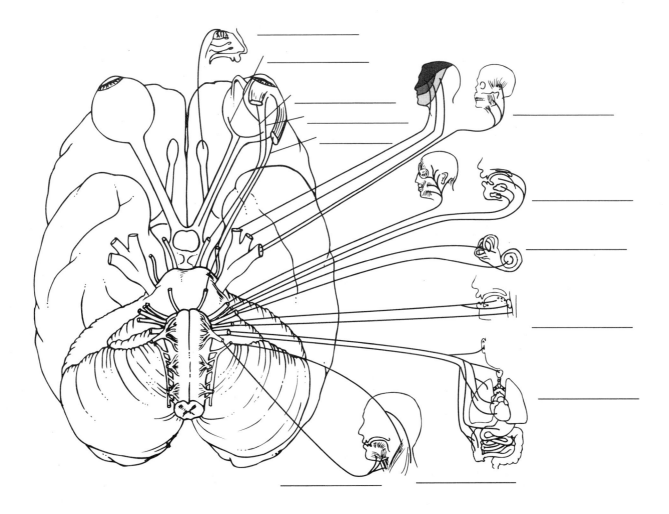

Fill in the name of each cranial nerve, then write S (sensory), M (motor), or MX (mixed)

REVIEW QUESTIONS

This test is for you and is intended to check your own mastery of the content. The answers are provided in Appendix A.

1. Prior to meeting a client for the first time, you review the medical record. The history and physical indicate that the client has an injury to Broca's area. When meeting this client you expect:

    a.   the client to have difficulty speaking.
    b.   receptive aphasia.
    c.   visual disturbances.
    d.   emotional lability.

2. The control of body temperature is located in:

    a.   Wernicke's area.
    b.   the thalamus.
    c.   the cerebellum.
    d.   the hypothalamus.

3. During the neurologic part of the assessment, the examiner wishes to test for stereognosis. The examiner would

    a.   have the client close his or her eyes, the examiner then raises the client's' arm and asks the client to describe its location.
    b.   touch the client with a tuning fork.
    c.   place a coin in the client's hand and ask him or her to identify it.
    d.   touch the client with a cold object.

4. During the examination of an infant, the examiner uses a cotton-tipped applicator to stimulate the anal sphincter of the child. The examiner does not observe a response. The examiner would note a lesion of:

    a.   L2.
    b.   T12.
    c   S2.
    d.   C5.

5. During a neurologic examination, the tendon reflex fails to appear. Before again striking the tendon, the examiner might use the technique of:

    a.   two-point discrimination.
    b.   reinforcement.
    c.   vibration.
    d.   graphesthesia.

6. Cerebellar function is assessed by which of the following tests?

    a.   Romberg
    b.   cranial nerve examination
    c.   coordination - hop on one foot
    d.   spinothalmic test

7. To elicit a Babinski response, the examiner:

    a.   gently taps the Achilles tendon.
    b.   strokes the lateral aspect of the sole of the foot from heel to the ball.
    c.   presents a noxious odor to a client.
    d.   observes the client walk heel to toe.

8. A positive Babinski is:

    a.   dorsiflexion of the big toe and fanning of all toes.
    b.   plantar flexion of the big toe with a fanning all toes.
    c.   the expected response in healthy adults.
    d.   withdrawal of the stimulated extremity from the stimulus.

9. The Cremasteric response:

    a.   is positive when disease of the pyramidal tract is present.
    b.   is positive when the ipsilateral testicle elevates upon stroking of the inner aspect of the thigh.
    c.   is a reflex of the receptors in the muscles of the abdomen.
    d.   is not a valid neurologic examination.

10. To examine for the function of the trigeminal nerve in an infant, the examiner would:

    a.   Startle the baby.
    b.   Hold an object within the child's line of vision.
    c.   Pinch the nose of the child.
    d.   Offer the baby a bottle.

11. Senile tremors may resemble parkinsonism, except that senile tremors do not include:

    a.   nodding the head as if responding yes or no.
    b.   rigidity and weakness of voluntary movement.
    c.   tremor of the hands.
    d.   tongue protrusion.

Match column A with column B

Column A—Cranial nerve	**Column B—Function**

Column A—Cranial nerve

12. ___   Olfactory

13. ___   Optic

14. ___   Oculomotor

15. ___   Trochlear.

16. ___   Trigeminal

17. ___   Abducens facial

18. ___   Acoustic

19. ___   Glossopharyngeal

20. ___   Vagus

21. ___   Spinal

22. ___   Hypoglossal

Column B—Function

a.   movement of the tongue

b.   vision

c.   lateral movement of the eye

d.   hearing and equilibrium

e.   talking, swallowing, carotid sinus, and carotid reflex

f.   smell

g.   extraocular movement, pupil constriction, down and inward movement of eye

h.   mastication and sensation of face, scalp, cornea

i.   phonation , swallowing, taste posterior 1/3 of tongue

j.   movement of trapezius and sternomastoid muscles

k.   down and inward movement of the eye.

l.   taste anterior 2/3 of tongue, close eyes

SKILLS LABORATORY/ CLINICAL SETTING

You are now ready for the clinical component of the neurologic system. The purpose of the clinical component is to practice the regional examination on a peer in the skills laboratory and to achieve the following:

Clinical Objectives

1. Demonstrate knowledge of the symptoms related to the neurologic system by obtaining a regional health history from a peer or client.

2. Demonstrate examination of the neurologic system by assessing the cranial nerves, cerebellar function, sensory system, motor system, and deep tendon reflexes.

3. Record the history and physical examination findings accurately, reach an assessment of the health state, and develop a plan of care.

Instructions

Gather all equipment for a complete neurologic examination. Wash your hands. Practice the steps of the exam on a peer or a client in the clinical setting, giving appropriate instructions as you proceed. Record your findings using the regional write-up sheet that follows. The first section is intended as a worksheet; the last page is intended for your narrative summary recording using the SOAP format.

REGIONAL WRITE-UP—NEUROLOGIC SYSTEM

Date _____

Client _____ Age ____ Sex ___ Occupation _____

Examiner _____

I. Health History

		No	Yes, explain
1.	Any unusually frequent or unusually severe **headaches**?	____	
2.	Ever had any **head injury**?	____	
3.	Ever feel **dizziness**?	____	
4.	Ever had any **convulsions**?	____	
5.	Any **tremors** in hands or face?	____	
6.	Any **weakness** in body part?	____	
7.	Any problem with **coordination**?	____	
8.	Any **numbness or tingling**?	____	
9.	Any problem **swallowing**?	____	
10.	Any problem **speaking**?	____	
11.	Past history of stroke, spinal cord injury, meningitis, congenital defect, alcoholism?	____	
12.	Any environmental/occupational hazards, e.g. insecticides?	____	

II. Physical Examination

A. Cranial nerves

I _____

II _____

III, IV, VI _____

V _____

VII _____

VIII _____

IX, X _____

XI _____

XII _____

B. Motor System

1. Muscles

 Size, strength, tone _____

 Involuntary movements _____

2. Cerebellar function

 Gait _____

 Romberg's test _____

 Rapid alternative movements _____

 Finger-to-finger test _____

 Finger-to-nose test _____

 Heel-to-shin test _____

C. Sensory System

1. Spinothalamic Tract

Pain _____

Temperature _____

Light touch _____

2. Posterior Column Tract

Vibration _____

Position (Kinesthesia) _____

Tactile Discrimination _____

Sterognosis _____

Graphesthesia _____

Two-point discrimination _____

D. Reflexes

	Bi	Tri	BR	P	A	PL($\downarrow$/$\uparrow$)	Abd	Cre	Bab
R									
L									

o = absent; 1+ = hypoactive; 2+ = normal; 3+ = hyperactive;
4+ = hyperactive with clonus; $\uparrow$ dorsiflexion; $\downarrow$ plantar flexion

REGIONAL WRITE-UP—NEUROLOGIC SYSTEM

Summarize your findings using the SOAP format.

Subjective (Client's reason for seeking care, health history)

Objective (Physical exam findings)   (Record reflexes on diagram below)

Assessment (Assessment of health state or problem, diagnosis)

Plan (Diagnostic evaluation, follow-up care, client teaching)

CHAPTER 22

Male Genitalia

Purpose: This chapter helps you to learn the structure and function of the male genitalia; to learn the methods of inspection and palpation of these structures; and to record the assessment accurately.

Reading Assignment: Jarvis, *Physical Examination and Health Assessment,* 2nd ed., Chapter 22, pp. 774-801

Audio-Visual Assignment: _____

Glossary: Study the following terms after completing the reading assignment. You should be able to cover the definition on the right and define the term out loud.

Chancre .... red, round, superficial ulcer with a yellowish serous discharge that is a sign of syphilis

Condylomata acuminata .... soft, pointed, fleshy papules that occur on the genitalia and are caused by the human papillomavirus (HPV)

Cryptorchidism .... undescended testes

Cystitis .... inflammation of the urinary bladder

Epididymis .... structure composed of coiled ducts located over the superior and posterior surface of the testes, which stores sperm

Epispadias .... congenital defect in which urethra opens on the dorsal (upper) side of penis instead of at the tip

Hernia .... weak spot in abdominal muscle wall (usually in area of inguinal canal or femoral canal) through which a loop of bowel may protrude

Herpes genitalis .... a sexually transmitted disease characterized by clusters of small painful vesicles, caused by a virus

Hydrocele .... cystic fluid in tunica vaginalis surrounding testis

Hypospadias .... congenital defect in which urethra opens on the ventral (under) side of penis rather than at the tip

Orchitis	acute inflammation of testis, usually associated with mumps
Paraphimosis	foreskin is retracted and fixed behind the glans penis
Peyronie's disease	nontender hard plaques on the surface of penis, associated with painful bending of penis during erection
Phimosis	foreskin is advanced and tightly fixed over the glans penis
Prepuce	(foreskin) the hood or flap of skin over the glans penis that often is surgically removed after birth by circumcision
Priapism	prolonged painful erection of penis without sexual desire
Spermatic cord	collection of vas deferens, blood vessels, lymphatics, and nerves that ascends along the testis and through the inguinal canal into the abdomen
Spermatocele	retention cyst in epididymis filled with milky fluid that contains sperm
Torsion	sudden twisting of spermatic cord; a surgical emergency
Varicocele	dilated tortuous varicose veins in the spermatic cord
Vas deferens	duct carrying sperm from the epididymis through the abdomen and then into the urethra

STUDY GUIDE

After completing the reading assignment and the audio-visual assignment, you should be able to answer the following questions in the spaced provided.

1. Describe the function of the cremaster muscle.

2. Identify the structures that provide transport of sperm.

3. Describe the significance of the inguinal canal and the femoral canal.

4. List the pros and cons of circumcision of the male newborn.

5. Discuss ways of creating an environment that will provide psychologic comfort for the client and examiner during the examination of male genitalia.

6. List teaching points to include with the client teaching of testicular self-examination.

7. Discuss the rationale for making certain that testes have descended in the male infant.

8. Contrast the physical appearance and clinical significance of these scrotal lumps:

   epididymitis

   varicocele

   spermatocele

   testicular tumor

   hydrocele

9. Contrast the anatomic course and the clinical significance of these hernias:

   indirect inguinal

   direct inguinal

   femoral

10. Fill in the labels indicated on the illustrations on the following page.

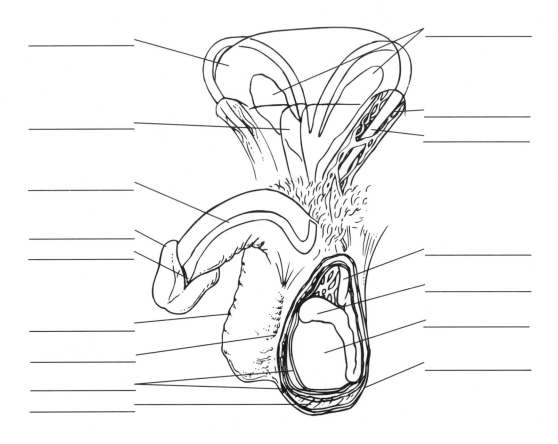

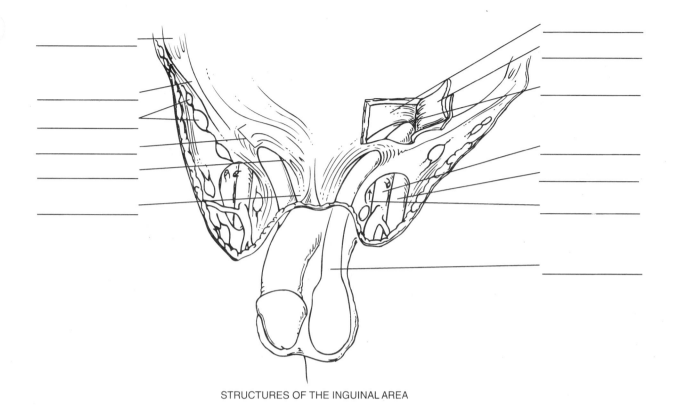

STRUCTURES OF THE INGUINAL AREA

REVIEW QUESTIONS

This test is for you and is intended to check your own mastery of the content. Answers are provided in Appendix A.

1. The examiner is going to inspect and palpate a male client for a hernia. During this exam, the client is instructed to:

   a. hold his breath during palpation.
   b. cough after the examiner has gently inserted the exam finger into the rectum.
   c. bear down when the examiner's finger is in the inguinal canal.
   d. relax in a supine position while the exam finger is inserted into the canal.

2. During inspection of the scrotum a normal finding would be:

   a. The testes are equal in size and hang evenly.
   b. The left testicle is larger than the right.
   c. The left testicle hangs lower than the right.
   d. The right testicle hangs lower than the left.

3. H. T. has come to the clinic for a follow-up visit. Six months ago, he was started on a new medication. The class of medication most likely to cause impotence and the side-effect therefore explored by the nurse is:

   a. antipyretics.
   b. bronchodilators.
   c. corticosteroids.
   d. antihypertensives.

4. Prostatic hypertrophy occurs frequently in older men. The symptoms that may indicate this problem are:

   a. polyuria and urgency.
   b. dysuria and oliguria.
   c. straining, loss of force and sense of residual urine.
   d. foul smelling urine and dysuria.

5. A 64-year-old man has come for a health examination. A normal age-related change in the scrotum would be:

   a. testicular atrophy.
   b. testicular hypertrophy.
   c. pendulous scrotum.
   d. increase in scrotal rugae.

6. During palpation of the testes, the normal finding would be:

   a. firm to hard, and rough.
   b. nodular.
   c. 2 to 3 cm long by 2 cm wide and firm.
   d. firm, rubbery, and smooth.

7. A 20-year-old man has indicated that he does not perform self testicular examination. One of the facts that should be shared with him is that testicular cancer occurs in men aged:

   a. under 15.
   b. 15 to 34.
   c. 35 to 55.
   d. 55 and older.

8. During the examination of a full term newborn male, a finding requiring investigation would be:

   a. absent testes.
   b. meatus centered at the tip of the penis.
   c. wrinkled scrotum.
   d. penis 2 to 3 cm in length.

9. During transillumination of a scrotum, a nontender mass is noted. This finding is suggestive of:

   a scrotal hernia.
   b. scrotal edema.
   c. orchitis.
   d. hydrocele.

10. Write a narrative account of an assessment of male genitalia with normal findings.

SKILLS LABORATORY/CLINICAL SETTING

You are now ready for the clinical component of the male genitalia exam. Because of the need to maintain personal privacy, it is likely you will not practice this examination on a classmate. Your practice likely will be with a teaching mannequin in the skills laboratory or with a client in the clinical setting. Before you proceed, discuss the feelings that may be experienced by client and examiner and methods to increase the comfort of both. Make sure you have discussed the steps of the examination with your instructor before examining a client.

Clinical Objectives

1. Demonstrate knowledge of the signs and symptoms related to the male genitalia by obtaining a pertinent health history.

2. Inspect and palpate the penis and scrotum.

3. Palpate the inguinal region for hernia.

4. Teach a testicular self-examination.

5. Record the history and physical examination findings accurately, reach an assessment of the health state, and develop a plan of care.

Instructions

Prepare the examination setting and gather your equipment. Wash your hands; wear gloves during the examination. Practice the steps of the exam on a client in the clinical setting, giving appropriate instructions as you proceed. Record your findings using the regional write-up sheet that follows. The front of the page is intended as a worksheet; the back of the page is intended for your narrative summary recording using the SOAP format.

NOTES

REGIONAL WRITE-UP—MALE GENITALIA

Date _____

Client _____ Age ____ Sex ___ Occupation _____

Examiner _____

I. Health History

	No	Yes, explain

1. Any urinary **frequency, urgency,** or wakening during night to urinate? _____ | _____

2. Any **pain** or **burning** with urinating? _____ | _____

3. Any **trouble starting urine stream**? _____ | _____

4. Urine **color cloudy** or **foul-smelling**? _____ | _____
    red-tinged or **bloody**? _____ | _____

5. Any **problem controlling your urine**? _____ | _____

6. Any **pain or sores** on penis? _____ | _____

7. Any **lump** in testicles or scrotum? _____ | _____
    Do you perform testicular self-exam? _____ | _____

8. In relationship now involving intercourse? _____ | _____
    Use a contraceptive? Which one? _____ | _____

9. Any contact with partner who has sexually transmitted disease? _____ | _____

II. Physical Examination

A. Inspect and palpate penis
Skin condition _____
Glans _____
Urethral meatus _____
Shaft _____

B. Inspect and palpate the scrotum
Skin condition _____
Testes _____
Spermatic cord _____
Transillumination (if indicated) _____

C. Inspect and palpate for hernia
Inguinal canal _____
Femoral area _____

D. Palpate inguinal lymph nodes
E. Teach testicular self-examination

REGIONAL WRITE-UP—MALE GENITALIA

Summarize your findings using the SOAP format.

Subjective (Client's reason for seeking care, health history)

Objective (Physical exam findings)

Assessment (Assessment of problem, diagnosis)

Plan (Diagnostic evaluation, follow-up care, client teaching)

PERFORMANCE CHECKLIST

TEACHING TESTICULAR SELF- EXAMINATION

	S	U	Comments
I. Cognitive			
1. Explain:			
a. Why testicles are examined			
b. who should perform TSE			
c. frequency of testicular exam			
2. Describe the technique			
II. Performance			
1. Explains to client need for TSE			
2. Instructs client on technique of TSE by:			
a. describing method of palpating testicles			
b. describing normal findings			
c. describing abnormal findings to look for			
3. Instructs client to report unusual findings promptly			

CHAPTER 23

Female Genitalia

Purpose: This chapter helps you to learn the structure and function of the female genitalia; the methods of inspection and palpation of the internal and external structures; the procedures for collection of cytological specimens; and to record the assessment accurately.

Reading Assignment: Jarvis, Physical Examination and Health Assessment, 2nd ed., Chapter 23, pp. 803 - 846.

_____

Audio-Visual Assignment: _____

_____

Glossary: Study the following terms after completing the reading assignment. You should be able to cover the definition on the right and define the term out loud.

Adnexa	accessory organs of the uterus, i.e., ovaries and fallopian tubes
Amenorrhea	absence of menstruation; termed secondary amenorrhea when menstruation has begun and then ceases, most common cause is pregnancy
Bartholin's glands	vestibular glands located on either side of the vaginal orifice, which secrete a clear lubricating mucus during intercourse
Bloody show	dislodging of thick cervical mucus plug at end of pregnancy, which is a sign of beginning of labor
Caruncle	small, deep red mass protruding from urethral meatus, usually due to urethritis
Chadwick's sign	bluish discoloration of cervix that occurs normally in pregnancy at 6 to 8 weeks' gestation
Chancre	red, round, superficial ulcer with a yellowish serous discharge that is a sign of syphilis

Clitoris	small, elongated, erectile tissue in the female, located at anterior juncture of labia minora
Cystocele	prolapse of urinary bladder and its vaginal mucosa into the vagina with straining or standing
Dysmenorrhea	abdominal cramping and pain associated with menstruation
Dyspareunia	painful intercourse
Dysuria	painful urination
Endometriosis	aberrant growths of endometrial tissue scattered throughout pelvis
Fibroid	(myoma) hard painless nodules in uterine wall that cause uterine enlargement
Gonorrhea	sexually transmitted disease characterized by purulent vaginal discharge, or may have no symptoms
Hegar's sign	softening of cervix that is a sign of pregnancy, occuring at 10 to 12 weeks' gestation
Hematuria	red-tinged or bloody urination
Hymen	membranous fold of tissue partly closing vaginal orifice
Leukorrhea	whitish or yellowish discharge from vaginal orifice
Menarche	onset of first menstruation usually between 11 to 13 years of age
Menopause	cessation of the menses, usually occurring around 48 to 51 years
Menorrhagia	excessively heavy menstrual flow
Multipara	condition of having two or more pregnancies
Nullipara	condition of first pregnancy
Papanicolaou test	painless test used to detect cervical cancer
Polyp	cervical polyp is bright red, soft, pedunculated growth emerging from os
Rectouterine pouch	(cul-de-sac of Douglas) deep recess formed by the peritoneum between the rectum and cervix
Rectocele	prolapse of rectum and its vaginal mucosa into vagina with straining or standing
Salpingitis	inflammation of fallopian tubes
Skene's glands	(paraurethral glands)
Vaginitis	inflammation of vagina
Vulva	external genitalia of female

STUDY GUIDE

After completing the reading assignment and the audio-visual assignment, you should be able to answer the following questions in the spaces provided.

1. List the external structures of the female genitalia.

2. Describe the size, shape, and location of the internal structures of the female genitalia.

3. Cite the physical changes in the uterus and cervix that are noted during pregnancy at:

    2 weeks' gestation _____

    4 - 6 weeks _____

    6 - 8 weeks _____

    8 - 12 weeks _____

    10 - 12 weeks _____

    20 - 24 weeks _____

    term _____

4. Outline the changes observed during the perimenopausal period.

5. Discuss ways of creating an environment that will provide psychologic comfort for both client and practitioner during the female genitalia examination.

6. Discuss selection, preparation, and insertion of the vaginal speculum.

7. Describe the appearance or sketch these normal variations of the cervix and os:

   nulliparous

   parous

   stellate lacerations

   cervical eversion

   nabothian cysts

8. List the steps in procedure of obtaining these specimens:

   endocervical specimen using cytobrush

   cervical scrape using spatula

   vaginal pool

9. When applying acetic acid (white vinegar) to the cervix and vaginal mucosa, list the normal response, and the response suggesting infection.

10. Discuss the procedure and rationale for bimanual examination and list normal findings for cervix, uterus, adnexa.

11. Discuss infection control precautions during examination of female genitalia and procuring of specimens.

12. Describe the appearance or sketch the appearance of the following abnormalities of the cervix:
    Chadwick's sign

    erosion

    polyp

    carcinoma

13. List the characteristics of vaginal discharge associated with the following conditions of vaginitis:

    candidiasis

    trichomoniasis

    bacterial vaginosis

    chlamydia

    gonorrhea

14. Differentiate the signs and symptoms of these conditions of adnexal enlargement:

    ectopic pregnancy

    ovarian cyst.

15. Fill in the labels indicated on the following illustrations.

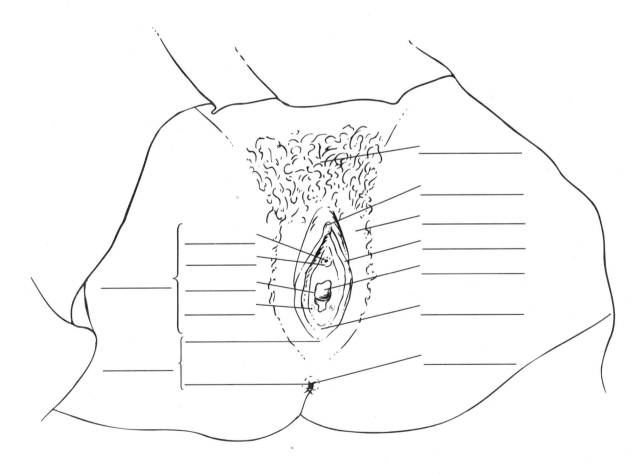

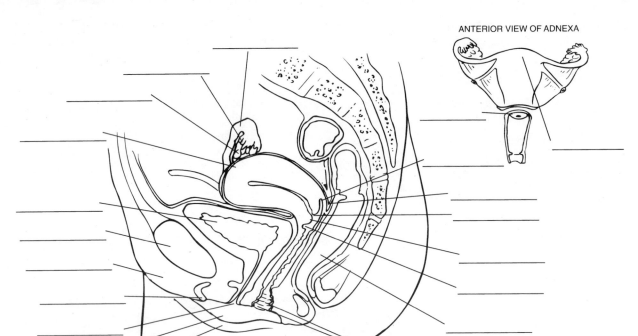

ANTERIOR VIEW OF ADNEXA

REVIEW QUESTIONS

This test is for you and is intended to check your own mastery of the content. Answers are provided in Appendix A.

1. Vaginal lubrication is provided during intercourse by:

   a. the labia minora.
   b. sebaceous follicles.
   c. Skene's glands.
   d. Bartholin's glands.

2. A young woman has come for her first gynecologic examination. Since she has not had any children, the examiner would expect the cervical os to appear:

   a. smooth and circular.
   b. irregular and slit like.
   c. irregular and circular.
   d. smooth and enlarged.

3. A client has come for an examination because of a missed menstrual period and a positive home pregnancy test. Examination reveals a cervix that appears cyanotic. This is referred to as:

   a. Goodell's sign
   b. Hegar's sign.
   c. Tanner's sign.
   d. Chadwick's sign.

4. During the examination of the genitalia of a 70-year-old female a normal finding would be:

   a. hypertrophy of the mons pubis.
   b. increase in vaginal secretions.
   c. thin and sparse pubic hair.
   d. bladder prolapse.

5. For a woman, history of her mother's health during pregnancy is important. A medication that requires frequent follow-up is:

   a. corticosteriod.
   b. theophylline.
   c. diethylstilbestrol.
   d. aminoglycoside.

6. A woman has come for health care complaining of a thick, white discharge with intense itching. These symptoms are suggestive of:

   a. atrophic vaginitis.
   b. trichomoniasis.
   c. chlamydia.
   d. candidiasis.

7. To prepare the vaginal speculum for insertion the examiner:

   a. lubricates it with a water soluble lubricant.
   b. lubricates it with petrolatum.
   c. warms it under the light, then inserts it into the vagina.
   d. lubricates it with warm water.

8. To insert the speculum as comfortably as possible, the examiner:

   a. opens the speculum slightly and inserts in an upward direction.
   b. presses the introitus down with one hand, inserts the blades obliquely with the other.
   c. spreads the labia with one hand, inserts the closed speculum horizontally with the other.
   d. pushes down on the introitus, inserts the speculum in an upward direction.

9. Before withdrawing the speculum, the examiner swabs the cervix with a swab soaked in acetic acid. This exam is done to assess for:

   a. herpes simplex virus.
   b. contact dermatitis.
   c. human papilloma virus.
   d. carcinoma.

10. Select the best description of the uterus.

    a. anteverted, round asymmetrical organ.
    b. a pear-shaped, thick-walled organ flattened anteroposteriorly.
    c. retroverted, almond-shaped asymmetrical organ.
    d. midposition, thick-walled oval organ.

11. A woman believed to be 28 weeks pregnant is being examined. The height of the fundus would be palpated at:

    a. the lower edge of the umbilicus.
    b. halfway between the umbilicus and xiphoid.
    c. almost to the xiphoid.
    d. halfway between the symphysis and umbilicus.

12. Write a narrative account of an assessment of female genitalia with normal findings.

SKILLS LABORATORY/ CLINICAL SETTING

You are now ready for the clinical component of the female genitalia exam. Because of the need to maintain personal privacy, it is likely you will not practice this examination on a peer. Your practice likely will be with a teaching mannequin in the skills laboratory or with a client in the clinical setting under the guidance of a preceptor. Before you proceed, discuss the feelings that may be experienced by client and examiner and methods to increase the comfort of both. With your instructor, discuss methods of positioning the client, steps in using the vaginal speculum, steps in procuring specimens, and methods of infection control precautions.

Clinical Objectives

1. Demonstrate knowledge of the signs and symptoms related to the female genitalia by obtaining a pertinent health history.

2. Demonstrate measures to increase client comfort before and during the examination.

3. Demonstrate knowledge of infection control precautions before, during and after the examination.

4. Inspect and palpate the external genitalia.

5. Using the vaginal speculum, gather materials for cytologic study.

6. Inspect and palpate the internal genitalia.

7. Record the history and physical examination findings accurately, reach an assessment of the health state, and develop a plan of care.

Instructions

Prepare the examination setting and gather your equipment. Collect the health history before the client disrobes for the examination. Wash your hands; wear gloves during the examination; wash hands again after removing gloves. Practice the steps of the exam on a client in the clinical setting, giving appropriate instructions as you proceed. Record your findings using the regional write-up sheet that follows. The first section is intended as a worksheet; the last page is intended for your narrative summary recording using the SOAP format. Collection of data for the rectal examination is usually combined with the examination of female genitalia; see Chapter 24 for the regional write-up sheet for the rectal exam.

REGIONAL WRITE-UP—FEMALE GENITALIA

Date _____

Client_____ Age____ Sex___ Occupation_____

Examiner_____

I. Health History

No   Yes, explain

1. Date of **last menstrual period**? _____
    Age at first period? Usual cycle? _____
    Duration? Usual amount of flow? _____
    Any pain or cramps with period? _____
2. Ever been **pregnant**? # times? _____
    Describe pregnancy (ies) _____
    Any complications? _____
3. Periods slowed down or **stopped**? _____
4. How often have **gyne. checkup**? _____
    Date of last Pap? Results? _____
5. Any problems with **urinating**? _____
6. Any unusual **vaginal discharge**? _____
7. **Sores** or **lesions** in genitals? _____
8. In relationship now involving intercourse? _____
9. Use a contraceptive? Which one? _____
10. Any contact with partner who has
    sexually transmitted disease? _____
11. Any precautions to reduce risk of STDs? _____
12. Taking any medications? _____
    Any hormone therapy? _____

II. Physical Examination

A. Inspect external genitalia
Skin color and characteristics _____
Hair distribution _____
Symmetry _____
Clitoris_____
Labia _____
Urethral opening _____
Vaginal opening _____
Perineum _____

B. Palpate external genitalia
Skene's glands _____
Bartholin's glands _____
Perineum _____
Assess perineal muscle strength _____
Assess for vaginal wall bulging or urinary incontinence _____
Discharge and characteristics _____

C. Speculum examination

    Inspect cervix and os

        Color _____

        Position _____

        Size _____

        Surface _____

        Discharge and characteristics _____

    Obtain cervical smears and cultures

        Endocervical specimen

        Cervical scrape

        Vaginal pool

        Other (if indicated)

    Complete acetic acid wash

    Inspect vaginal wall as speculum is removed

D. Bimanual examination

    Cervix

        Consistency _____

        Mobility _____

        Tenderness with motion _____

    Uterus

        Size and shape _____

        Consistency _____

        Position _____

        Mobility _____

        Tenderness _____

    Adnexa

        Able to palpate? (Be honest) _____

        Size and shape of ovaries _____

        Tenderness _____

        Masses _____

    Rectovaginal examination

REGIONAL WRITE-UP—FEMALE GENITALIA

Summarize your findings using the SOAP format.

Subjective (Client's reason for seeking care, health history)

Objective (Physical exam findings)   Record findings on diagram below

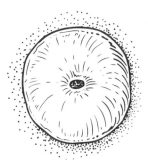

Assessment (Assessment of health state or problem, diagnosis)

Plan (Diagnostic evaluation, follow-up care, client teaching)

Anus, Rectum, and Prostate

Purpose: This chapter helps you to learn the structure and function of the anus and rectum and the male prostate gland; the methods of inspection and palpation of these structures; and how to record the assessment accurately.

Reading Assignment: Jarvis, *Physical Examination and Health Assessment,* 2nd ed.,

Chapter 24, pp. 848–862.

_____

Audio-Visual Assignment: _____

_____

Glossary: Study the following terms after completing the reading assignment. You should be able to cover the definition on the right and define the term out loud.

Fissure	painful longitudinal tear in tissue, e.g., in the superficial mucosa at the anal margin
Hemorrhoid	flabby papules of skin or mucous membrane in the anal region caused by a varicose vein of the hemorrhoidal plexus
Melena	blood in the stool
Pruritus	itching or burning sensation in the skin
Steatorrhea	excessive fat in the stool as in gastrointestinal malabsorption of fat
Valves of Houston	one of three semilunar transverse folds that cross one-half the circumference of the rectal lumen

STUDY GUIDE

After completing the reading assignment and the audio-visual assignment, you should be able to answer the following questions in the spaces provided.

1. State the length of the anal canal and the rectum in the adult, and describe the location of these structures in the lower abdomen.

2. Describe the size, shape, and location of the male prostate gland.

3. List a few examples of high-fiber foods of the soluble type, and of the insoluble type; what advantages do these foods have for the body?

4. List screening measures that are recommended for early detection of colon/rectal cancer; of prostate cancer.

5. State the method of promoting anal sphincter relaxation in order to aid palpation of the anus and rectum.

6. Describe the normal physical characteristics of the prostate gland that would be assessed by palpation:

   size

   shape

   surface

   consistency

   mobility

   sensitivity

7. Describe the physical appearance and clinical significance of pilonidal cyst, and anorectal fistula.

8. Define the condition *benign prostatic hypertrophy*, list the usual symptoms the man experiences with this condition, and describe the physical characteristics.

9. Fill in the labels indicated on the following illustration.

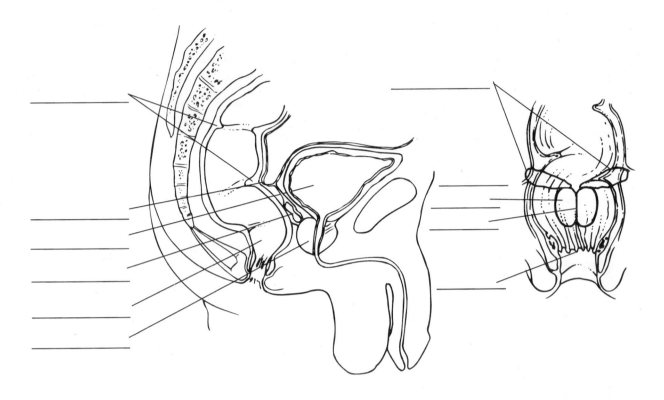

REVIEW QUESTIONS

This test is for you and is intended to check your own mastery of the content. Answers are provided in Appendix A.

1. The gastrocolic reflex is :

   a. a peristaltic wave.
   b. the passage of meconium in the newborn.
   c. another term for Borborygmi.
   d. reverse peristalsis.

2. The incidence of benign prostatic hypertrophy (BPH) is highest among:

   a. Euro-Americans.
   b. Afro-Americans.
   c. Hispanics.
   d. Asians.

3. Select the best description of the anal canal.

   a. A 12 cm long portion of the large intestine
   b. Under involuntary control of the parasym-pathetic nervous system
   c. A 3.8 cm long outlet of the gastrointestinal tract
   d. An S-shaped portion of the colon

4. While good nutrition is important for everyone, foods believed to help certain gastrointestinal disorders are:

   a. high in fiber.
   b. low in fat.
   c. high in protein.
   d. high in carbohydrate.

5. Select the position that is least desirable for examination of the rectum.

   a. standing
   b. lithotomy
   c. squatting
   d. prone

6. The bulbourethral gland is assessed:

   a. during an examination of a female patient.
   b. during an examination both male and female patients.
   c. during an examination of a male patient.
   d. cannot be assessed with a rectal examination

7. Inspection of stool is an important part of the anal examination. Normal stool is:

   a. Black in color and tarry in consistency.
   b. Brown in color and soft in consistency.
   c. Clay colored and dry in consistency.
   d. Varies depending upon the individuals' diet.

8. Write a narrative account of a rectal assessment with normal findings.

SKILLS LABORATORY/CLINICAL SETTING

You are now ready for the clinical component of the rectal examination. This regional examination usually is combined with the examination of the male genitalia or with examination of the female genitalia.

Clinical Objectives

1. Demonstrate knowledge of the signs and symptoms related to the rectal area by obtaining a pertinent health history.

2. Inspect and palpate the perianal region.

3. Test any stool specimen for occult blood.

4. Record the history and physical examination findings accurately.

Instructions

Prepare the examination setting and gather your equipment. Wash your hands; wear gloves during the examination; wash hands again after removing gloves. Practice the steps of the exam on a client in the clinical setting, giving appropriate instructions as you proceed. Record your findings using the regional write-up sheet that follows. Note that only the worksheet is included in this chapter. Your narrative summary recording using the SOAP format can be included with the narrative summary of the genitalia.

NOTES

REGIONAL WRITE-UP—ANUS, RECTUM, AND PROSTATE GLAND Date _____

Client_____ Age ____ Sex ___ Occupation _____

Examiner_____

I. Health History

	No	Yes, explain
1. Bowels move **regularly**? How often? Usual color? Hard or soft?	_____	_____
2. Any **change** in usual bowel habits?	_____	_____
3. Ever had **black or bloody stool**?	_____	_____
4. Take any medications?	_____	_____
5. Any **rectal itching, pain, or hemorrhoids?**	_____	_____
6. Any family history of **colon/rectal polyps or cancer**?	_____	_____
7. Describe usual amount high fiber foods in diet?		_____

II. Physical Examination

A. Inspect the perianal area
Skin condition _____
Sacrococcygeal area _____
Note skin integrity while client performs Valsalva maneuver _____

B. Palpate anus and rectum
Anal sphincter _____
Anal canal _____
Rectal wall _____
Prostate gland (for males)
    Size _____
    Shape _____
    Surface _____
    Consistency _____
    Mobility _____
    Any tenderness _____
Cervix (for females) _____

C. Examination of stool
Visual inspection _____
Test for occult blood _____

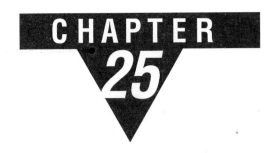

The Complete Health Assessment: Putting it all Together

Purpose: This chapter helps you to learn the methods of integrating the regional examinations so that you will be able to conduct a complete physical examination on a well young adult.

Reading Assignment: Jarvis, *Physical Examination and Health Assessment,* 2nd ed., Chapter 25, pp. 866–887.

Clinical Objectives

1. Demonstrate skills of inspection, percussion, palpation, and auscultation.

2. Demonstrate correct use of instruments, including assembly, manipulation of component parts, and positioning with client.

3. Use appropriate terminology and correctly pronounce medical terminology with clinical instructor and with client.

4. Choreograph the complete examination in a systematic manner, including integration of certain regional assessments throughout the examination (e.g. skin, musculoskeletal).

5. Coordinate procedures to limit position changes for examiner and client.

6. Describe accurately the findings of the examination, including normal and abnormal findings.

7. Demonstrate appropriate infection control measures.

8. Recognize and maintain the privacy and dignity of the client.

    a.   Adequately explain what is being done, while limiting smalltalk.
    b.   Consider client's anxiety and fears.
    c.   Consider your own facial expression and comments.
    d.   Demonstrate confidence, empathy, and gentle manner.
    e.   Acknowledge and apologize for any discomfort caused.
    f.   Provide for privacy and warmth at all times.
    g.   Determine comfort level, pausing if client becomes tired.
    h.   Wash hands and don gloves appropriately.
    i.   Allow adequate time for each step.
    j.   Briefly summarize findings to client, and thank client for his or her time.

Instructions

The key to success in this venture is practice; you should conduct at least three complete physical examination practices in your preparation for this final examination proficiency. You are responsible for obtaining a peer "client" for the examination. You should prepare your own note card "outline" for the examination. You may refer to this minimally during the examination, but over dependence on your notes will constitute failure. You will have 45 minutes in which to conduct the examination (not including setup, or genitalia examinaiton). If you practice three times, you will have no difficulty completing the examination in the alloted time.

Prepare the examination setting. Arrange for proper lighting. If you are using a hospital bed instead of an examination table, make sure to adjust the bed height during the exam to allow for your own visualization of the client, and for the client's ease in getting into and out of the bed. Arrange adequate client gown, bath blankets, and drapes.

Gather your equipment. The following items are needed for a complete physical examination, including female genitalia. Check with your clinical instructor for any items that you may omit for your own examination proficiency.

Platform scale with height attachment
Skinfold calipers
Sphygmomanometer with appropriate size cuff
Stethoscope with bell and diaphragm endpieces
Thermometer
Flashlight or penlight
Otoscope/ophthalmoscope
Tuning fork
Nasal speculum
Tongue depressor
Pocket vision screener
Skin-marking pen
Flexible tape measure and ruler marked in centimeters
Reflex hammer
Sharp object (sterile needle or split tongue blade)
Cotton balls
Bivalve vaginal speculum
Disposible gloves
Materials for cytologic study
Lubricant
Fecal occult blood test materials

Record your findings using the writeup sheets that follow. Your clinical instructor may ask you to record your findings ahead of time, following one of your practice sessions. Then you can give your writeup to the instructor to follow along as you perform the final examination proficiency.
Good luck!

COMPLETE PHYSICAL EXAMINATION

Date _____

Client_____ Age _____ Sex ___ Occupation _____

Examiner_____

General Survey of Client

1. Appears stated age _____

2. Level of consciousness _____

3. Skin color _____

4. Nutritional status _____

5. Posture and position _____

6. Obvious physical deformities _____

7. Mobility: gait, use of assistive devices, ROM of joints, no involuntary movement

   _____

8. Facial expression _____

9. Mood and affect _____

10. Speech: articulation, pattern, content appropriate, native language

    _____

11. Hearing_____

12. Personal hygiene_____

Measurement and Vital Signs

1. Weight _____

2. Height _____

3. Skinfold thickness, if indicated_ _____

4. Vision using Snellen eye chart _____

   OD_____ OS_____ Correction?_____

5. Radial pulse, rate and rhythm _____

6. Respirations, rate, depth _____

7. Blood pressure

   Right arm _____ (sitting or lying?)

   Left arm _____ (sitting or lying?)

8. Temperature (if indicated) _____

STAND IN FRONT OF CLIENT, CLIENT IS SITTING

Skin

1. Hands and nails _____

2. (For rest of exam, examine skin with corresponding region)

   Color and pigmentation _____

   Temperature _____

   Moisture _____

Texture _____

Turgor _____

Any lesions _____

Head and Face

1. Scalp, hair, cranium _____

2. Face (cranial nerve VII) _____

3. Temporal artery, temporomandibular joint _____

4. Maxillary sinuses, frontal sinuses _____

Eyes

1. Visual fields (cranial nerve II) _____

2. Extraocular muscles, corneal light reflex _____

   Cardinal positions of gaze (cranial nerves III, IV, VI) _____

3. External structures _____

4. Conjunctivae _____

   Sclerae _____

   Corneas _____

   Irides _____

5. Pupils _____

6. Ophthlamoscope, red reflex _____

   Disc _____

   Vessels _____

   Retinal background _____

Ears

1. External ear _____

2. Any tenderness _____

3. Otoscope, ear canal _____

   Tympanic membrane _____

4. Test hearing (cranial nerve VIII), voice test _____

   Weber test _____

   Rinne test _____

Nose

1. External nose _____

2. Patency of nostrils _____

3. Speculum, nasal mucosa _____

   Septum _____

   Turbinates _____

Mouth and Throat

1. Lips and buccal mucosa _____

   Teeth and gums _____

   Tongue _____

   Hard/soft palate _____

2. Tonsils _____

3. Uvula (cranial nerves IX, X) _____

4. Tongue (cranial nerve XII) _____

Neck

1. Symmetry, lumps, pulsations _____

2. Cervical lymph nodes _____

3. Carotid pulse (bruits if indicated) _____

4. Trachea _____

5. ROM and muscle strength (cranial nerve XI) _____

MOVE TO BACK OF CLIENT, CLIENT SITTING

6. Thyroid gland _____

Chest and Lungs, Posterior and Lateral

1. Thoracic cage configuration _____

   Skin characteristics _____

   Symmetry _____

2. Symmetric expansion _____

   Tactile fremitus _____

   Lumps or tenderness _____

3. Spinous processes _____

4. Percussion over lung fields _____

   Diaphragmatic excursion _____

5. CVA tenderness _____

6. Breath sounds _____

7. Adventitious sounds _____

MOVE TO FRONT OF CLIENT

Chest and Lungs, Anterior

1. Respirations and skin characteristics _____

2. Tactile fremitus, lumps, tenderness _____

3. Percuss lung fields _____

4. Breath sounds _____

Upper extremities

1. ROM and muscle strength _____

2. Epitrochlear nodes _____

Breasts

1. Symmetry, mobility, dimpling _____
2. Supraclavicular and infraclavicular areas _____

CLIENT SUPINE, STAND AT CLIENT'S RIGHT

3. Breast palpation _____
4. Nipple _____
5. Axillae and regional nodes _____
6. Teach breast self-examination _____

Neck vessels

1. Jugular venous pulse _____
2. Jugular venous pressure, if indicated _____

Heart

1. Precordium, pulsations and heave _____
2. Apical impulse _____
3. Precordium, thrills _____
4. Apical rate and rhythm _____
5. Heart sounds _____

Abdomen

1. Contour, symmetry _____
   Skin characteristics _____
   Umbilicus and pulsations _____
2. Bowel sounds _____
3. Vascular sounds _____
4. Percussion _____
5. Liver span in right MCL _____
6. Spleen _____
7. Light and deep palpation _____
8. Palpation of liver, spleen, kidneys, aorta _____
9. Abdominal reflexes, if indicated _____

Inguinal Area

1. Femoral pulse _____
2. Inguinal nodes _____

Lower Extremities

1. Symmetry _____
   Skin characteristics, hair distribution _____

2. Pulses, popliteal _____

   Posterior tibial _____

   Dorsalis pedis _____

3. Temperature, pretibial edema _____

4. Toes _____

CLIENT SITS UP

5. ROM and muscle strength, Hips _____

   Knees _____

   Ankles and feet _____

Neurologic

1. Sensation, Face _____

   Arms and hands _____

   Legs and feet _____

2. Position sense _____

3. Sterognosis _____

4. Cerebellar function, finger-to-nose _____

5. Cerebellar function, heel-to-shin _____

6. Deep tendon reflexes

   Biceps_____   Triceps _____

   Brachioradialis_____   Patellar _____

   Achilles _____

7. Babinski reflex _____

CLIENT STANDS UP

Musculoskeletal

1. Walk across room _____

   Walk, heel to toe _____

2. Walk on tiptoes, then walk on heels _____

3. Romberg sign _____

4. Shallow knee bend _____

5. Touch toes _____

6. ROM of spine _____

Male Genitalia

1. Penis and scrotum _____

2. Testes and spermatic cord _____

3. Inguinal hernia _____

4. Teach testicular self examination _____

Male Rectum

1. Perianal area _____

2. Rectal walls and prostate gland _____

3. Stool for occult blood _____

FEMALE CLIENT IN LITHOTOMY POSITION
Female Genitalia and Rectum

1. Perineal and perianal areas _____

2. Vaginal speculum, cervix and vaginal walls _____

3. Procure specimens _____

4. Bimanual, cervix, uterus, adnexa _____

   _____

5. Rectovaginal _____

6. Stool for occult blood _____

HELP CLIENT SIT UP

THANK CLIENT FOR TIME, DEPART FROM CLIENT

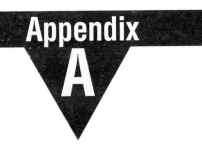

Appendix A

Answers to Review Questions

Chapter 1

1. a
2. d
3. c
4. b
5. c
6. a
7. In addition to accurate diagnosis and treatment of illness, health care must address the mind, body, and spirit as interdependent and functioning as a whole within the environment. A list of assessment factors nurses use to judge has been identified by the American Nurses' Association. Assessment is the collection of those data that relate to the health state of the client. the information gathered during the assessment process forms the data base. The extent of data collected depends upon the clinical situation. The four types of data bases are complete, episodic, follow-up, and emergency. A diagnosis is made based on the information in the data base. Nursing disgnoses are the common language with which nurses communicate their findings. The frequency of visits to the health practitioner is determined by the health needs and age group of the client.

Chapter 2

1. c
2. b
3. a
4. d
5. c
6. b
7. d
8. c
9. b
10. d
11. b

Chapter 3

1. b
2. c
3. a
4. c
5. b
6. a

Chapter 4

1. a
2. b
3. b
4. c
5. d
6. b
7. a
8. d
9. b
10. d
11. b

Chapter 5

1. d
2. a
3. c
4. b
5. a
6. c
7. c
8. a
9. b
10. d

Chapter 6

1. d
2. a
3. d
4. c
5. b
6. c
7. b
8. c
9. a
10. c
11. i
12. d
13. b
14. g
15. f
16. a
17. e
18. h
19. Client is dressed and groomed appropriately for season and setting. Posture is erect, with no involuntary body movements. Oriented to time person and place. Recent and remote memory intact. Affect and verbal responses appropriate. Perceptions and thought processes logical and coherent.

Chapter 7

1. c
2. d
3. c
4. c
5. c
6. b
7. b
8. a
9. a
10. c
11. c
12. d

Chapter 8

1. d
2. c
3. b
4. a
5. c
6. d
7. c
8. c

Chapter 9

1. d
2. c
3. b
4. a
5. c
6. a
7. b
8. b
9.
10. a
11. d

Chapter 10

1. b
2. d
3. a
4. d
5. b
6. d
7. c
8. c
9. a
10. a
11. c
12. b
13. b
14. a
15. a
16. b
17. c
18. a
19. b
20. d
21. b
22. a
23. g
24. c
25. f
26. d
27. e

Chapter 11

1. d
2. a
3. b
4. a
5. d
6. d
7. c
8. c
9. e
10. f
11. h
12. g
13. i
14. j
15. b
16. d
17. a
18. a

Chapter 12

1. b
2. c
3. a
4. b
5. d
6. c
7. a
8. c
9. a
10. Instruct the client to hold the head steady and follow the examiner's finger. The examiner holds the finger 12 inches from the individual and moves it clockwise to the positions of 2, 3, 4, and 8, 9, and 10 o'clock and back to the center each time. A normal response is parallel tracking of the object with both eyes.

Chapter 13

1. c
2. a
3. d
4. b
5. a
6. c
7. c
8. d

Chapter 14

1. c
2. d
3. d
4. a
5. b
6. a
7. b
8. d
9. c

Chapter 15

1. d
2. b
3. a
4. c
5. b
6. c
7. c
8. c
9. b
10. d

Chapter 16

1. a
2. b
3. b
4. a
5. c
6. b
7. b
8. d
9. c
10. d
11. b
12. e
13. a
14. c
15. d
16. b
17. e
18. a
19. d
20. f
21. c
22. b

Chapter 17

1. c
2. b
3. c
4. b
5. d
6. d
7. b
8. b
9. a
10. a
11. e
12. c
13. f
14. a
15. b
16. d

17. Liver to RA via inferior vena cava, through tricuspid valve to right ventricle, through the pulmonic valve to the pulmonary artery, picks up oxygen in the lungs, returns to LA, to LV via mitral valve, through aortic valve to aorta and out to the body.

18. The major risk factors for heart disease and stroke are hypertension, smoking, high cholesterol levels, obesity and diabetes. In addition, the use of oral contraceptives and lack of post-menopausal endogenous estrogen may be risk factors for some women.

Chapter 18

1. a
2. c
3. c
4. b
5. c
6. d
7. a
8. d
9. b

Chapter 19

1. c
2. c
3. a
4. d
5. c
6. a
7. d
8. d
9. d
10. a
11. d
12. a
13. c
14. b

Chapter 20

1. d
2. b
3. d
4. c
5. d
6. a
7. a
8. c
9. b
10. The musculoskeletal system provides support to stand erect and the ability to move. The system protects inner organs, produces red blood cells and provides for the storage of minerals.
11. b
12. e
13. g
14. i
15. d
16. a
17. j
18. m
19. k
20. n
21. l
22. h
23. f
24. c

Chapter 21

1. a.
2. d
3. c
4. c
5. b
6. c
7. b
8. a
9. b
10. d
11. b
12. f
13. b
14. g
15. k
16. h
17. c
18. d
19. i
20. e
21. j
22. a

Chapter 22

1. c
2. c
3. d
4. c
5. c
6. d
7. b
8. a
9. d
10. Voids clear, amber urine 5 to 6 times a day. No nocturia, dysuria or hesitancy. No pain or discharge from penis. Sexually active with multiple partners. Uses prophylaxis that is satisfactory for both partners. No history of sesually transmitted disease. No lesions, inflammation or discharge from penis noted on examination. Testes descended without masses. No inguinal hernia.

Chapter 23

1. d
2. a
3. d
4. c
5. d
6. d
7. d
8. b
9. c
10. b
11. b
12. Menarche at age 14, cycle 28 to 32 days of 4–5 days duration. Flow moderate with no dysmenorrhea. Gravida 0/Para 0/Ab 0. Has annual Gyn exam. No urinary problems, no vaginal discharge. Uses barrier method of birth control. Method satisfactory to self and partner.

Chapter 24

1. a
2. b
3. c
4. a
5. d.
6. c
7. b
8. No recent change in bowel habits. One BM daily, soft, dark brown in color. No pain or bleeding. No medications. Diet includes 4 servings of fruits and vegetables daily. No hemorrhoids or rectal lesions noted. Sphincter tone good. No masses or tenderness on palpation. No masses, tenderness or enlargement of prostate. Stool is Hematest negative.

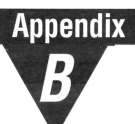

Appendix B

Summary of Infant Growth and Development

AGE (MOS)	PHYSICAL COMPETENCY	INTELLECTUAL COMPETENCY	EMOTIONAL-SOCIAL COMPETENCY
1 to 2	Holds head in alignment when prone; Moro reflex to loud sound; follows objects; smiles	Reflex activity; vowel sounds produced	Gratification through sucking and basic needs being promptly met; smiles at people
2 to 4	Turns back to side; raises head and chest 45–90 degrees off bed and supports weight on arms; reaches for objects; follows object through midline; drools; begins to localize sounds; prefers configuration of face	Reproduces behavior initially achieved by random activity; imitates behavior previously done. Visually studies objects; locates sounds; makes cooing sounds; does not look for objects removed from presence	Social responsiveness; awareness of those who are not primary care giver; smiles in response to familiar face
4 to 6	Birth weight doubled; teeth eruption may begin; sits with stable head and back control; rolls from abdomen to back; picks up object with palmar grasp	Some intentional actions; some sense of object permanence, looks on same path for vanished object; recognizes partially hidden objects; more systematic in imitative behavior; babbles	Prefers primary care giver; sucking needs decrease; laughs in pleasure
6 to 8	Turns back to stomach; sits alone; crawls; transfers objects hand to hand; turns to sound behind	Continued development as in 4 to 6 months	Differentiated response to nonprimary care takers; evidence of "stranger" or "separation" anxiety
8 to 10	Creeps; pulls to stand; pincer grasp	Actions more goal directed; able to solve simple problems by using previously mastered responses. Actively searches for an object that disappears	Attachment process complete
10 to 12	Birth weight tripled; cruises; stands by self; may use spoon	Begins to imitate behavior done before by others but not by self. Understands words being said; may say 1 to 4 words. Intentionality is present	Begins to explore and separate briefly from parent

	NUTRITION	PLAY	SAFETY
1 to 2	Breastfed or fortified formula	Variety of positions. Care taker should hold and talk to infant, large, brightly colored objects	Car carrier; proper use of infant seat
2 to 4	As for 1 to 2 months	Talk to and hold. Musical toys; rattle, mobile. Variety of objects of different color, size and texture; mirror, crib toys, variety of settings	Do not leave unattended on couch, bed, etc. Remove any small objects that infant could choke on
4 to 6	Introduction of solids; initial store of iron depletion	Talk and hold. Provide open space to move and objects to grasp	Keep environment free of safety hazards; check toys for sharp edges and small pieces that might break
6 to 8	As for 4 to 6 months	Provide place to explore. Stack toys, blocks; nursery rhymes	Check infant's expanding environment for hazards
8 to 10	As for 4 to 6 months	Games: hide and seek; peek-a-boo, pat-a-cake, looking at pictures in a book	Keep: electrical outlets plugged, cords out of reach, stairs blocked, coffee and end tables cleared of hazards. Do not leave alone in bathtub. Keep poisons out of reach and locked up. Continue use of safety seat in car
10 to 12	More solids than liquids; increasing use of cup; begin to wean	Increase space; read to infant. Name and point to body parts. Water; sand play; ball	As for 8 to 10 months

(Modified from Betz C, Hunsberger M, Wright S; Family-Centered Nursing Care of Children, 2nd ed. Philadelphia, WB Saunders, 1994, pp 148–149. Used with permission.)

Appendix C

Summary of Toddler Growth and Development and Health Maintenance

AGE	PHYSICAL COMPETENCY	INTELLECTUAL COMPETENCY	EMOTIONAL-SOCIAL COMPETENCY

General:
1 to 3 yrs
	Gains 5 kg (11 lb).
	Grows 20.3 cm (8 in).
	12 teeth erupt
	Nutritional requirements:
	  Energy 100 Kcal/kg/day
	  Fluid 115–125 ml/kg/day
	  Protein 1.8 gm/kg/day
	  See Chapter 6 for vitamins and
	  minerals.
		Learns by exploring and experimenting
		Learns by imitating. Progresses from a
		vocabulary of three to four words at
		12 months to about 900 words at 36
		months.
			Central crisis: to gain a sense of auton-
			omy versus doubt and shame. Demon-
			strates independent behaviors. Exhi-
			bits attachment behavior strongly and
			regularly until third birthday. Fears
			persist of strange people, objects, and
			places and of aloneness and being aban-
			doned. Egocentric in play (parallel play).
			Imitation of parents in household tasks
			and activities of daily living.

15 mos	Legs appear bowed. Walks alone, climbs, slides downstairs backward. Stacks two blocks. Scribbles spontaneously. Grasps spoon but rotates it, holds cup with both hands. Takes off socks and shoes.	Trial and error method of learning. Experiments to see what will happen. Says at least three words. Uses expressive jargon.	Shows independence by trying to feed self and helps in undressing.
18 mos	Runs but still falls. Walks upstairs with help. Slides downstairs backwards. Stacks three to four blocks. Clumsily throws a ball. Unzips a large zipper. Takes off simple garments.	Begins to maintain a mental image of an absent object. Concept of object permanence fully develops. Has vocabulary of 10 or more words. Holophrastic speech (one word used to communicate whole ideas)	Fears the water. Temper tantrums may begin. Negativism and dawdling predominate. Bedtime rituals begin. Awareness of gender identity begins. Helps with undressing.
24 mos	Runs quickly and with fewer falls. Pulls toys and walks sideways. Walks downstairs hanging on a rail (does not alternate feet). Stacks six blocks. Turns pages of a book. Imitates vertical and circular strokes. Uses spoon with little spilling. Can feed self. Puts on simple garments. Can turn door knobs.	Enters into preconceptual phase of preoperational period: Symbolic thinking and symbolic play. Egocentric thinking, imagination, and pretending are common. Has vocabulary of about 300 words. Uses two-word sentences (telegraphic speech). Engages in monologue.	Fears the dark and animals. Temper tantrums may continue. Negativism and dawdling continue. Bedtime rituals continue. Sleep resisted overtly. Usual- ly shows readiness to begin bowel and bladder control. Explores genitalia. Brushes teeth with help. Helps with dressing and undressing.
36 mos	Has set of deciduous teeth at about 30 months. Walks downstairs alternating feet. Rides tricycle. Walks with balance and runs well. Stacks eight to ten blocks. Can pour from a pitcher. Feeds self completely. Dresses self almost com- pletely (does not know front from back). Cannot tie shoes.	Preconceptual phase of preoperational period as for 24 months. Uses around 900 words. Constructs complete sentences and uses all parts of speech.	Temper tantrums subside. Negativism and dawdling subside. Bedtime rituals subside. Self-care in feeding, elimination and dressing enhances self-esteem.

Appendix continues on following page

(From Betz C, Hunsberger M, Wright S; Family-Centered Nursing Care of Children, 2nd ed. Philadelphia, WB Saunders, 1994, pp 190–191. Used with permission.)

	NUTRITION	PLAY	SAFETY
General: 1 to 3 yrs	Milk 16–24 oz. Appetite decreases. Wants to feed self. Has food jags. Never force food; give nutritious snacks. Give iron and vitamin supplementation only if poor intake.	Books at all stages. Needs physical and quiet activities, does not need expensive toys.	Never leave alone in tub. Keep poisons, including detergents and cleaning products, out of reach. Use car seat. Have ipecac in house.
15 mos	Vulnerable to iron deficiency anemia. Give table foods except for tough meat and hard vegetables. Wants to feed self.	Stuffed animals, dolls, music toys. Peek-a-boo, hide and seek. Water and sand play. Stacking toys. Roll ball on floor. Push toys on floor. Read to toddler.	Keep small items off floor (pins, buttons, clips). Child may choke on hard food. Cords and tablecloths are a danger. Keep electrical outlets plugged and poisons locked away. Risk of kitchen accidents with toddler under foot.
18 mos	Negativism may interfere with eating. Encourage self-feeding. Is easily distracted while eating. May play with food. High activity level interferes with eating.	Rocking horse. Nesting toys. Shape-sorting cube. Pencil or crayon. Pull toys. Four-wheeled toy to ride. Throw ball. Running and chasing games. Rough-housing. Puzzles. Blocks. Hammer and peg board.	Falls: from riding toy in bathtub from running too fast Climbs up to get dangerous objects. Keep dangerous things out of waste-basket.
24 mos	Requests certain foods; therefore snacks should be controlled. Imitates eating habits of others. May still play with food and especially with utensils and dish (pouring, stacking).	Clay and Play-Doh. Finger paint. Brush paint. Record player with record and story book and songs to sing along. Toys to take apart. Toy tea sets. Puppets. Puzzles.	May fall from outdoor large play equipment. Can reach farther than expected (knives, razors, and matches must be kept out of reach).
36 mos	Sits in booster seat rather than high chair. Verbal about likes and dislikes.	Likes playing with other children, building toys, drawing and painting, doing puzzles. Imitation household objects for doll play. Nurse and doctor kits. Carpenter kits.	Protect from: turning on hot water falling from tricycle striking matches.

(From Betz C, Hunsberger M, Wright S; Family-Centered Nursing Care of Children, 2nd ed. Philadelphia, WB Saunders, 1994, pp 190–191. Used with permission.)

Appendix D

Growth, Development, and Health Promotion for Preschoolers

AGE (YRS)	PHYSICAL COMPETENCY	INTELLECTUAL COMPETENCY	EMOTIONAL-SOCIAL COMPETENCY
General: 3 to 5	Gains 4.5 kg (10 lb) Grows 15 cm (6 in) 20 teeth present Nutritional requirements: 　Energy: 1250 to 1600 cal/day (or 90 to 100 Kcal/kg/day) 　Fluid: 100 to 125 ml/kg/day 　Protein: 30 g/day (or 3 g/kg/day) 　Iron: 10 mg/day	Becomes increasingly aware of self and others Vocabulary increases from 900 to 2100 words Piaget's preoperational/intuitive period	Freud's phallic stage 　Oedipus complex—boy 　Electra complex—girl Erikson's stage of Initiative vs. Guilt
3	Runs, stops suddenly Walks backward Climbs steps Jumps Pedals tricycle Undresses self Unbuttons front buttons Feeds self well	Knows own sex Desires to please Sense of humor Language—900 words Follows simple direction Uses plurals Names figure in picture Uses adjectives/adverbs	Shifts between reality and imagination Bedtime rituals Negativism decreases Animism and realism: anything that moves is alive
4	Runs well, skips clumsily Hops on one foot Heel-toe walk Up and down steps without holding rail Jumps well Dresses and undresses Buttons well, needs help with zippers, bows Brushes teeth Bathes self Draws with some form and meaning	More aware of others Uses alibis to excuse behavior Bossy Language—1500 words Talks in sentences Knows nursery rhymes Counts to 5 Highly imaginative Name calling	Focuses on present Egocentrism/ unable to see the viewpoint of others, unable to understand another's inability to see own viewpoint Does not comprehend anticipatory explanation Sexual curiosity Oedipus complex Electra complex
5	Runs skillfully Jumps 3–4 steps Jumps rope, hops, skips Begins dance Roller skates Dresses without assistance Tie shoelaces Hits nail on head with hammer Draws person—6 parts Prints first name	Aware of cultural differences Knows name and address More independent More sensible/less imaginative Copies triangle, draws rectangle Knows four or more colors Language—2100 words, meaningful sentences Understands kinship Counts to 10	Continues in egocentrism Fantasy and daydreams Resolution of Oedipus/Electra complex, girls identify with mother, boys with father Body image and body boundary especially important in illness Shows tension in nail-biting, nose-picking, whining, snuffling

Appendix continues on following page

(From Betz C, Hunsberger M, Wright S; Family-Centered Nursing Care of Children, 2nd ed. Philadelphia, WB Saunders, 1994, pp 235–236. Used with permission.)

	NUTRITION	PLAY	SAFETY
General: 3 to 5	Carbohydrate intake approximately 40 to 50 percent of calories Good food sources of essential vitamins and minerals Regular tooth brushing Parents are seen as examples; if parent won't eat it, child won't	Reading books is important at all ages Balance highly physical activities with quiet times Quiet rest period takes the place of nap time Provide sturdy play materials	Never leave alone in bath or swimming pool Keep poisons in locked cupboard; learn what household things are poisonous Use car seats and seatbelts Never leave child alone in car Remove doors from abandoned and refrigerators
3	1250 cal/day Due to increased sex identity and imitation, copies parents at table and will eat what they eat Different colors and shapes of foods can increase interest	Participates in simple games Cooperates, takes turns Plays with group Uses scissors, paper Likes crayons, coloring books Enjoys being read to and "reading" Plays "dress-up" and "house" Likes fire engines	Teach safety habits early Let water out of bathtub; don't stand in tub Caution against climbing in unsafe areas, onto or under cars, unsafe buildings, drainage pipes Insist on seatbelts worn at all times in cars
4	Good nutrition 1400 cal/day Nutritious between-meal snacks essential Emphasis on quality not quantity of food eaten Mealtime should be enjoyable, not for criticism As dexterity improves, neatness increases	Longer attention span with group activities "Dress-up" with more dramatic play Draws, pounds, paints Likes to make paper chains, sewing cards Scrapbooks Likes being read to, records, and rhythmic play "Helps" adults	Teach to stay out of streets, alleys Continually teach safety; child understands Teach how to handle scissors Teach what are poisons and why to avoid Never allow child to stand in moving car
5	Good nutrition 1600 cal/day Encourage regular tooth brushing Encourage quiet time before meals Can learn to cut own meal Frequent illnesses from increased exposure increases nutritional needs	Plays with trucks, cars, soldiers, dolls Likes simple games with letters or numbers Much gross motor activity: water, mud snow, leaves, rocks Matching picture games	Teach child how to cross streets safely Teach child not to speak to strangers or get into cars of strangers Insist on seatbelts Teach child to swim

(From Betz C, Hunsberger M, Wright S; Family-Centered Nursing Care of Children, 2nd ed. Philadelphia, WB Saunders, 1994, pp 235–236. Used with permission.)

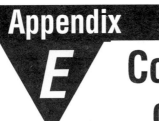

Appendix E
Competency Development of the School-Aged Child

AGE (YRS)	PHYSICAL COMPETENCY	INTELLECTUAL COMPETENCY	EMOTIONAL-SOCIAL COMPETENCY
General: 6 to 12	Gains an average of 2.5 to 3.2 kg/year (5 ¹/₂ to 7 lbs/year. Overall height gains of 5.5 cm (2 in) per year; growth occurs in spurts and is mainly in trunk and extremities. Loses deciduous teeth; most of permanent teeth erupt. Progressively more coordinated in both gross and fine motor skills. Caloric needs increase with growth spurts.	Masters concrete operations. Moves from egocentrism; learns he or she is not always right. Learns grammar and expression of emotions and thoughts. Vocabulary increases to 3000 words or more; handles complex sentences.	Central crisis: industry vs. inferiority; wants to do and make things. Progressive sex education needed. Wants to be like friends; competition important. Fears body mutilation, alterations in body image; earlier phobias may recur, nightmares; fears death. Nervous habits common.
6 to 7	Gross motor skill exceeds fine motor coordination. Balance and rhythm are good—runs, skips, jumps, climbs, gallops. Throws and catches ball. Dresses self with little or no help.	Vocabulary of 2500 words. Learning to read and print; beginning concrete concepts of numbers, general classification of items. Knows concepts of right and left; morning, afternoon, and evening; coinage. Intuitive thought process. Verbally aggressive, bossy, opinionated, argumentative. Likes simple games with basic rules.	Boisterous, outgoing, and a know-it-all, whiney; parents should sidestep power struggles, offer choices. Becomes quiet and reflective during seventh year; very sensitive. Can use telephone. Likes to make things: starts many, finishes few. Give some responsibility for household duties.
8 to 10	Myopia may appear. Secondary sex characteristics begin in girls. Hand-eye coordination and fine motor skills well established. Movements are graceful, coordinated. Cares for own physical needs completely. Constantly on move; plays and works hard; enforce balance in rest and activity.	Learning correct grammar and to express feelings in words. Likes books he or she can read alone; will read funny papers, scan newspaper. Enjoys making detailed drawings. Mastering classification, seriation, spatial and temporal, numerical concepts. Uses language as a tool; likes riddles, jokes, chants, word games. Rules guiding force in life now. Very interested in how things work, what and how weather, seasons, etc., are made.	Strong preference for same-sex peers; antagonizes opposite-sex peers. Self-assured and pragmatic at home; questions parental values and ideas. Has a strong sense of humor. Enjoys clubs, group projects, outings, large groups, camp. Modesty about own body increases over time; sex conscious. Works diligently to perfect skills he or she does best. Happy, cooperative, relaxed, and casual in relationships. Increasingly courteous and well-mannered with adults. Gang stage at a peak; secret codes and rituals prevail. Responds better to suggestion than dictatorial approach.
11 to 12	Vital signs approximate adult norms. Growth spurt for girls; inequalities between sexes are increasingly noticeable; boys greater physical strength. Eruption of permanent teeth complete except for third molars. Secondary sex characteristics begin in boys. Menstruation may begin.	Able to think about social problems and prejudices; sees others' points of view. Enjoys reading mysteries, love stories. Begins playing with abstract ideas. Interested in whys of health measures and understands human reproduction. Very moralistic; religious commitment often made during this time.	Intense team loyalty; boys begin teasing girls and girls flirt with boys for attention; best friend period. Wants unreasonable independence. Rebellious about routine; wide mood swings; needs some time daily for privacy. Very critical of own work. Hero worship prevails. "Facts of life" chats with friends prevail; masturbation increases. Appears under constant tension.

Appendix continued on following page

(From Betz C, Hunsberger M, Wright S; Family-Centered Nursing Care of Children, 2nd ed. Philadelphia, WB Saunders, 1994, pp 281–282. Used with permission.)

	NUTRITION	PLAY	SAFETY
General: 6 to 12	Fluctuations in appetite due to uneven growth pattern and tendency to get involved in activities. Tendency to neglect breakfast owing to rush of getting to school. Though school lunch is provided in most schools, child does not always eat it.	Plays in groups, mostly of same sex; "gang" activities predominate. Books for all ages. Bicycles important. Sports equipment. Cards, board and table games. Most of play is active games requiring little or no equipment.	Enforce continued use of safety belts during car travel. Bicycle safety must be taught and enforced. Teach safety related to hobbies, handicrafts, mechanical equipment.
6 to 7	Preschool food dislikes persist. Tendency for deficiencies in iron, vitamin A, and riboflavin. 100 ml/kg of water per day. 3 gm/kg protein daily.	Still enjoys dolls, cars and trucks. Plays well alone but enjoys small groups of both sexes; begins to prefer same sex peer during 7th year. Ready to learn how to ride a bicycle. Prefers imaginary, dramatic play with real costumes. Begins collecting for quantity, not quality. Enjoys active games such as hide-and-seek, tag, jumprope, roller skating, kickball. Ready for lessons in dancing, gymnastics, music. Restrict TV time to 1–2 hours/day.	Teach and reinforce traffic safety. Still needs adult supervision of play. Teach to avoid strangers, never take anything from strangers. Teach illness prevention and reinforce continued practice of other health habits. Restrict bicycle use to home ground; no traffic areas; teach bicycle safety. Teach the harmful use of drugs, alcohol, smoking. Set a good example.
8 to 10	Needs about 2100 calories/day; nutritious snacks. Tends to be too busy to bother to eat. Tendency for deficiencies in calcium, iron, and thiamine. Problem of obesity may begin now. Good table manners. Able to help with food preparation.	Likes hiking, sports. Enjoys cooking, woodworking, crafts. Enjoys cards and table games. Likes radio and records. Begins qualitative collecting now. Continue restriction on TV time.	Stress safety with firearms. Keep them out of reach and allow use only with adult supervision. Know who the child's friends are; parents should still have some control over friend selection. Teach water safety; swimming should be supervised by an adult
11 to 12	Male needs 2500 calories per day; female needs 2250 (70 cal/kg/day). 75 ml/kg of water per day. 2 gm/kg protein daily.	Enjoys projects and working with hands. Likes to do errands and jobs to earn money. Very involved in sports, dancing, talking on phone. Enjoys all aspects of acting and drama.	Continue monitoring friends; Stress bicycle safety on streets and in traffic.

(From Betz C, Hunsberger M, Wright S; Family-Centered Nursing Care of Children, 2nd ed. Philadelphia, WB Saunders, 1994, pp 281–282. Used with permission.)

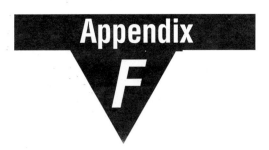

Appendix F

Characteristics of Adolescents

EARLY ADOLESCENCE (12 TO 14 YR)	MIDDLE ADOLESCENCE (15 TO 16 YR)	LATE ADOLESCENCE (17 TO 21 YR)
Becomes comfortable with own body; egocentric	"Tries out" adult-like behavior	Aware of own strengths and limitations; establishes own value system
Difficulty solving problems; thinks in present; cannot use past experience to control behavior; sense of invulnerability—society's rules do not apply to him or her	Begins to solve problems, analyze, and abstract	Able to verbalize conceptually: deals with abstract moral concepts; makes decisions re future
Struggle between dependent and independent behavior; begins forming peer alliance	Established peer group alliance with associated risk-taking behavior	Peer group diminishes in importance; may develop first intimate relationship
Parent-child conflict begins; teen argues but without logic	Peak turmoil in child-family relations; able to debate issues and use some logic but not continuously	Turbulence subsides. May move away from home. More adult-like friendship with parents

(From Foster R, Hunsberger M, Anderson JJ: Family-Centered Nursing Care of Children. Philadelphia, WB Saunders, 1989, p 359. Used with permission.)